SOMATIC EXERCISES FOR BEGINNERS

A 28-Day WAVE REVOLUTION to Defeat Stress, Relieve Difficult Emotions & Reconnect Body-Mind in less than 10 min/day | REAL PHOTOS + 60 VIDEOS step-by-step AUDIO guided

BONUS 1: ULTRA HD VIDEO COURSE | STEP-BY-STEP AUDIO GUIDED

BONUS 2: 28 DAY-Plan

BONUS 3: Somatics Plan Tracking Journal

BONUS 4: Nutrition and Fueling Your Success

BONUS 5: Meal Plan

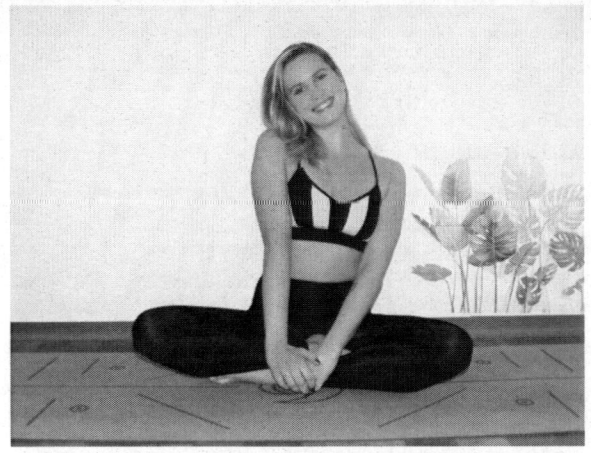

ALICIA DIAMOND

Table of Contents

INTRODUCTION

About me

I was born into a wonderful American family in Washington, the third of three siblings, with two exceptional parents.

As a girl, I was always into sports, and since I was little, I attended many fitness classes.

I had a serene and happy adolescence, crowned by a beautiful love story.

After 4 years of true love, just when I was about to get married, my boyfriend left me, and I began to experience my first panic attacks.

The final blow came a few months later when my father passed away: since then, I fell into depression, completely stopped exercising, gained over 40 pounds, and hardly ever left the house because I felt ugly and afraid of being around people.

I didn't want to be happy anymore, and I'm not ashamed to say that I had frequent suicidal thoughts.

I owe it to my friends who slowly pushed me to come out of it; I owe it to them that I'm still here.

I started practicing Pilates first, and in a few months, I managed to regain my former shape.

Then I discovered Yoga and Somatic exercises, which were a turning point for me: I gradually regained confidence in myself, felt better, panic attacks decreased until they disappeared, and I healed from all the traumas I had carried for so long.

Now, on the threshold of 40, after 15 years and more of practice and teaching, I have decided to help all the people who, like me, have suffered because we all deserve to be well!

"Somatic Exercises for Beginners," my second book after "Wall Pilates Workouts for Women," is dedicated to all the women who, like me, have suffered and want to defeat stress, relieve anxiety and chronic pain, manage difficult emotions, and lose weight.

My Mission

My mission is to help women of all ages and fitness levels. With 'Wall Pilates Workouts for Women,' I focused on strengthening muscle tone and losing weight with simple exercises suitable for everyone.

With my second book, 'Somatic Exercises for Women,' I aim to help all women heal from trauma, overcome panic attacks, defeat overstress, and naturally lose weight.

At the end of my structured 28-Day journey, all women will look in the mirror and say, 'I feel really different, I am much happier, I feel better, and I want to enjoy life!'

AUDIO-VIDEOS and 28-Day Journey

Why audio videos? All my books come with exclusive bonus audio videos. After years of experience, I'm convinced that videos with step-by-step audio instructions are incredibly helpful for beginners in mastering the proposed exercises.

I want nothing but the best for my readers through an:

All-in-One REAL PHOTOS Book+ Ultra HD VIDEO COURSE step-by-step AUDIO guided + 28-DAY journey!

Whether you're a seasoned fitness practitioner or stepping into this world for the first time, this workbook is designed to meet you where you are and accompany you on your Somatic journey.

I would also take the opportunity to remind that your honest and opened review on Amazon would be truly invaluable. Reader opinions like yours not only help me grow as an author but also assist other readers in their choice. Below the link to leave the review:

https://www.amazon.com/review/create-review/?asin=B0CWBJDQ5B

For any feedback or info, please do not hesitate to send me an email at aliciadiamond.fitness@gmail.com

With enthusiasm and dedication,

Alicia.

Chapter 1: Discovering Somatic Exercises

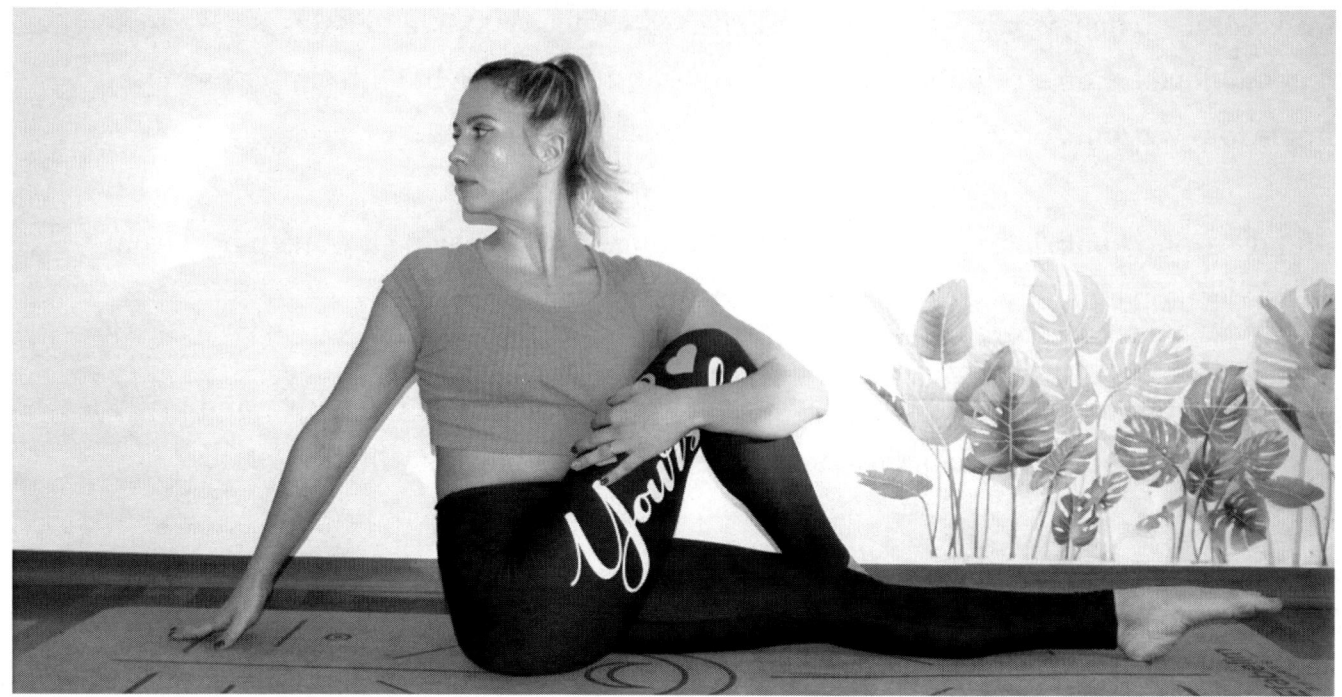

The Origins of Somatics: A Fusion of Tradition and Innovation

Somatics, as a field of study and practice, was developed by Thomas Hanna in the 20th century. Thomas Hanna, a philosopher and movement therapist, coined the term "somatics" to describe the study of the body as perceived from within. Hanna's work and the development of somatic practices can be traced back to the mid-20th century, and he founded the field of Hanna Somatic Education (HSE). Hanna's seminal book "Somatics: Reawakening The Mind's Control Of Movement, Flexibility, And Health" was published in 1988. While Hanna played a significant role in popularizing somatics, it's essential to note that various somatic approaches and methods have emerged over the years.

Somatics draws inspiration not only from modern Western practices but also from ancient Eastern philosophies. Concepts from tai chi and qi gong, with their emphasis on the flow of energy within the body, have significantly influenced the development of somatic practices. Over the last five decades, somatics has evolved into a profound discipline, blending traditional wisdom with contemporary understanding.

Somatic Exercises

The most common types of somatic exercises are:

1. **Hanna Somatics:** Developed by Thomas Hanna, this method emphasizes sensory motor awareness to release involuntary muscle contractions (sensory motor amnesia) through slow and controlled movements.

2. **Feldenkrais Method:** Created by Moshe Feldenkrais, this approach uses gentle movements and focused attention to improve movement patterns, flexibility, and coordination. It often involves both passive and active exploration of various body movements.

3. **Alexander Technique:** The Alexander Technique focuses on improving posture and movement by releasing tension and promoting efficient use of the body. It involves re-education of the mind-body connection to achieve better alignment and coordination.

4. **Body-Mind Centering (BMC):** Developed by Bonnie Bainbridge Cohen, BMC explores the relationship between the body and mind through movement and touch. It incorporates developmental movement patterns and focuses on embodying different systems within the body.

5. **Laban Movement Analysis:** Created by Rudolf Laban, this system provides a framework for understanding and analyzing movement. It includes exercises that promote awareness of the body in motion, exploring elements like space, weight, time, and flow.

6. **Continuum Movement:** Emilie Conrad developed Continuum Movement, which involves fluid and breath-based movements. Practitioners explore various ways of moving to enhance flexibility, release tension, and connect with the body's inherent wisdom.

7. **Body Awareness in Action (B.A.N.A.):** This approach combines elements of various somatic practices and mindfulness to increase body awareness and facilitate self-discovery. It often involves gentle movements, breathwork, and meditation.

8. **Somatic Yoga:** Somatic yoga integrates somatic principles into traditional yoga practices, emphasizing internal awareness, mindful movement, and releasing tension through slow, controlled poses.

9. **Mindful Movement Practices:** Mindfulness-based movement practices, such as Tai Chi and Qigong, focus on cultivating awareness of the body in motion. These practices often include slow, deliberate movements, breathwork, and meditation.

10. **Embodyoga:** Developed by Patty Townsend, Embodyoga combines traditional yoga with principles from somatics to deepen the practitioner's awareness of their body and enhance the mind-body connection.

Main Benefit of Somatics

Somatics is a field that encompasses various practices and therapeutic approaches aimed at enhancing bodily awareness and promoting overall well-being. It involves mindful movement and exercises designed to address and release chronic muscular tension, improve posture, and foster a deeper connection between the mind and body.

Somatic practices typically focus on the internal experience of movement, encouraging individuals to explore and understand their unique bodily sensations.

The goal is to:

- release patterns of tension, stress, and chronic muscle tension
- relieve pain developed due to past TRAUMA or habitual movements
- improve posture
- enhance overall well-being.

Key elements of Somatics include:

1. **Mind-Body Connection:** Somatics emphasizes the intricate connection between the mind and body. It recognizes that physical and emotional experiences are intertwined, and addressing both aspects is essential for holistic well-being.

2. **Awareness Through Movement:** Somatic exercises often involve slow, deliberate movements. Practitioners pay close attention to bodily sensations, encouraging a heightened awareness of how the body moves and feels.

3. **Release of Tension:** Somatics seeks to release chronic muscular tension by promoting relaxation and improved movement patterns. This can contribute to reduced pain, improved flexibility, and enhanced overall mobility.

4. **Integration of Breath:** Breath awareness is often integrated into somatic practices. Conscious breathing is used to promote relaxation, reduce stress, and deepen the mind-body connection.

5. **Exploration of Patterns:** Individuals engage in somatic exercises to explore and change movement patterns that may be contributing to discomfort or limitations. This process involves a mindful investigation into one's habitual ways of moving and holding tension.

6. **Enhanced Emotional Awareness:** Advocates of somatic therapies endorse the approach as **an** effective means of navigating repressed or blocked emotions stemming from traumatic experiences. Studies on   experiencing, a type of somatic therapy, demonstrated potential in

addressing negative emotional effects and trauma symptoms persisting over extended periods.

7. **Pain Relief:** Gentle somatic exercises, by directing attention to areas of injury or discomfort, offer insights into modifying movement, posture, and body language for pain reduction.

8. **Enhanced Mobility:** Somatic practices demonstrate promise in enhancing balance, coordination, and range of movement, particularly among older adults.

In conclusion, **Somatic is a Holistic Approach** to well-being, considering physical, emotional, and mental aspects. It is not solely focused on addressing symptoms but aims to promote overall health and resilience.

Somatic practice: Recommendations and Contraindications

Practice recommendations: Creating a conducive environment for somatics workouts is crucial for a fulfilling and effective experience. Here are some recommendations to prepare your environment for somatic practices:

1. **Quiet and Calm Space:** Choose a quiet and calm space for your somatics workouts. Minimize external distractions and noise to help you focus on the subtleties of movement and enhance your mindful awareness.

2. **Comfortable Flooring:** Opt for a comfortable and supportive flooring surface. Mats or carpets can provide the necessary cushioning for lying down or sitting during exercises. Ensure that the surface is clean and free from obstacles.

3. **Appropriate Lighting:** Ensure the lighting in your space is gentle and conducive to relaxation. Natural light is ideal, but if practicing in the evening, consider using soft, warm-toned artificial lighting to create a calming atmosphere.

4. **Comfortable Clothing:** Wear comfortable, loose-fitting clothing that allows for unrestricted movement. This enhances your ability to engage in the exercises without any constraints.

5. **Temperature Control:** Maintain a comfortable room temperature. You may want to have a blanket or extra layers nearby in case you feel chilly during relaxation or stillness exercises.

6. **Mindful Props:** Depending on the somatic practice you choose, consider having props such as a yoga block, blanket, or small pillow. These props can support your body and ensure that you maintain proper alignment during exercises.

7. **Personalized Music or Silence:** Choose whether you prefer to practice in silence or with soft, soothing music. Some individuals find that music enhances their experience, while others prefer the quiet for deeper concentration. Tailor the auditory environment to suit your preferences.

8. **Uninterrupted Time:** Set aside a dedicated time for your somatics workouts where you won't be interrupted. This allows you to fully engage in the practice without time constraints or external pressures.

9. **Digital Detox:** Consider turning off or silencing electronic devices to minimize distractions. This practice encourages a break from the demands of technology and fosters a more mindful and present workout.

10. **Personalized Aromatherapy:** Incorporate aromatherapy if it enhances your relaxation. Scented candles, essential oils, or incense can contribute to creating a calming ambiance.

11. **Visual Appeal:** Arrange your space with elements that bring you peace and joy. This could include plants, artwork, or other items that create a visually pleasing and positive atmosphere.

By thoughtfully preparing your environment, you create a supportive space that complements the goals of somatic practices—promoting relaxation, heightened awareness, and overall well-being. Remember, the goal is to tailor your environment to maximize your comfort and enhance the effectiveness of your somatics workouts.

Potential contraindications: individuals recovering from recent surgeries or injuries should seek clearance from healthcare professionals before engaging in somatic exercises, as well as those with unmanaged chronic health conditions, such as severe arthritis, osteoporosis, cardiovascular issues, or high blood pressure.

Pregnant women with complications or high-risk pregnancies should avoid certain movements and consult healthcare providers before practicing Somatics

Chapter 2: Somatic Exercises for Release Trauma

Some somatic exercises are specifically designed to release trauma because trauma can often manifest physically in the body as tension, stress, or other physical sensations. These exercises aim to address the physiological aspects of trauma by promoting relaxation, releasing stored tension, and restoring a sense of safety and control in the body. By engaging in somatic exercises tailored to trauma release, you can gradually process and release the physical manifestations of trauma, leading to greater emotional and psychological well-being.

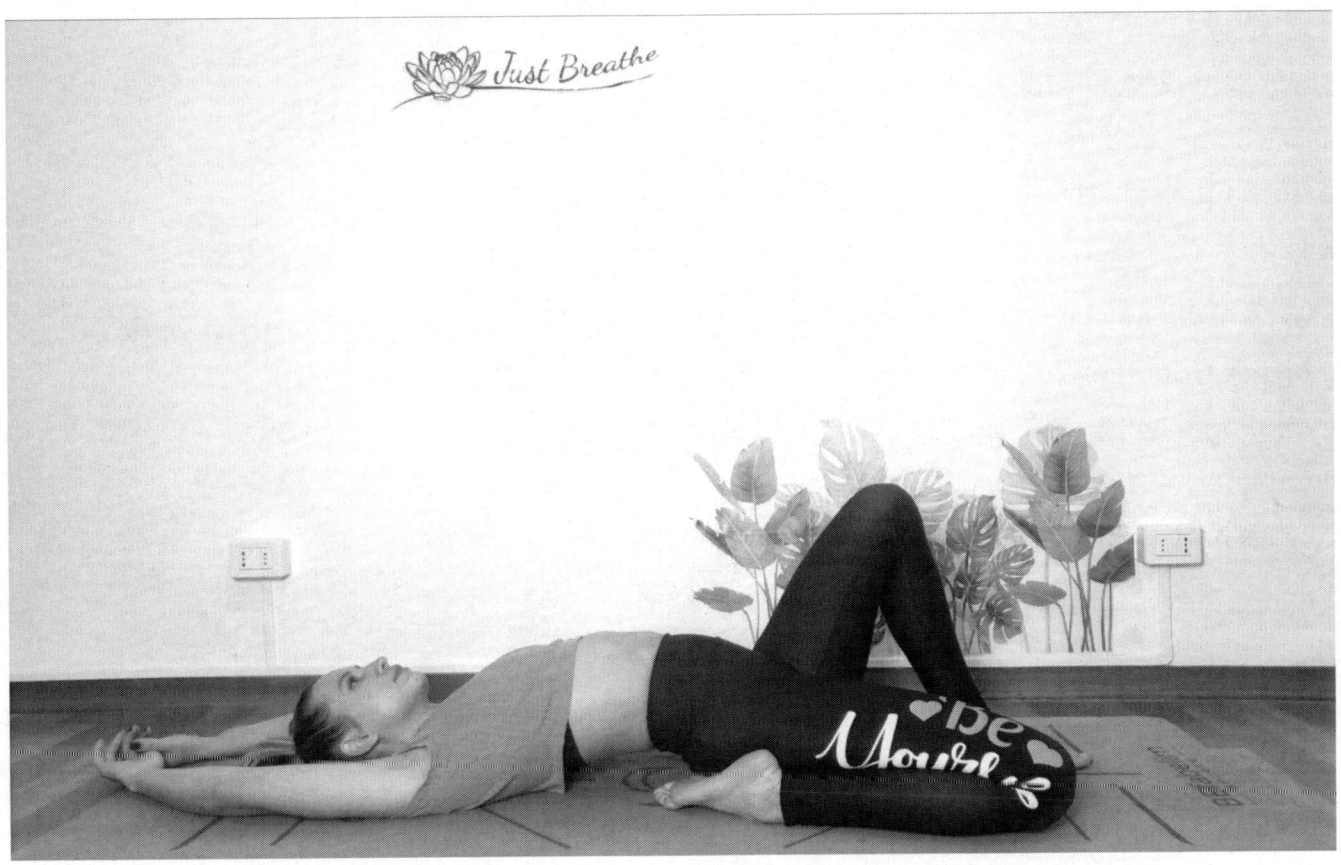

Release Trauma: Exercise 1

Benefits

Trauma often manifests as tension and holding patterns in the body. This first exercise helps to release physical tension, allowing you to let go of the physiological effects of trauma.

Instructions

1. Lie down on your back, knees bent and feet hip distance apart. Arms open wide with your palms facing up

2. Slowly, allow your knees to fall open as far as it's comfortable for you. When you get to the end, bring the soles of your feet together.

3. Slowly bring up your knees together about 2 inches from the ground. Take a pause here. You may be shaking, which is completely normal: It's a part of their release process.

4. Allow your knees to slowly drop back open. Bring your knees back together, another 2 inches closer. You may shake even more this time.

5. Slowly bring your knees back together and your feet flat on the floor.

Breathing

Inhale and Exhale as your knees slowly drop back open.

Inhale before bringing your knees back together.

Exhale as your bring your knees back and your feet flat on the floor.

Exhale to lift up the knee.

Repetitions, Sets, and Rest

5 repetitions, resting for 30 seconds each set.

Suitable for

Trauma Release.

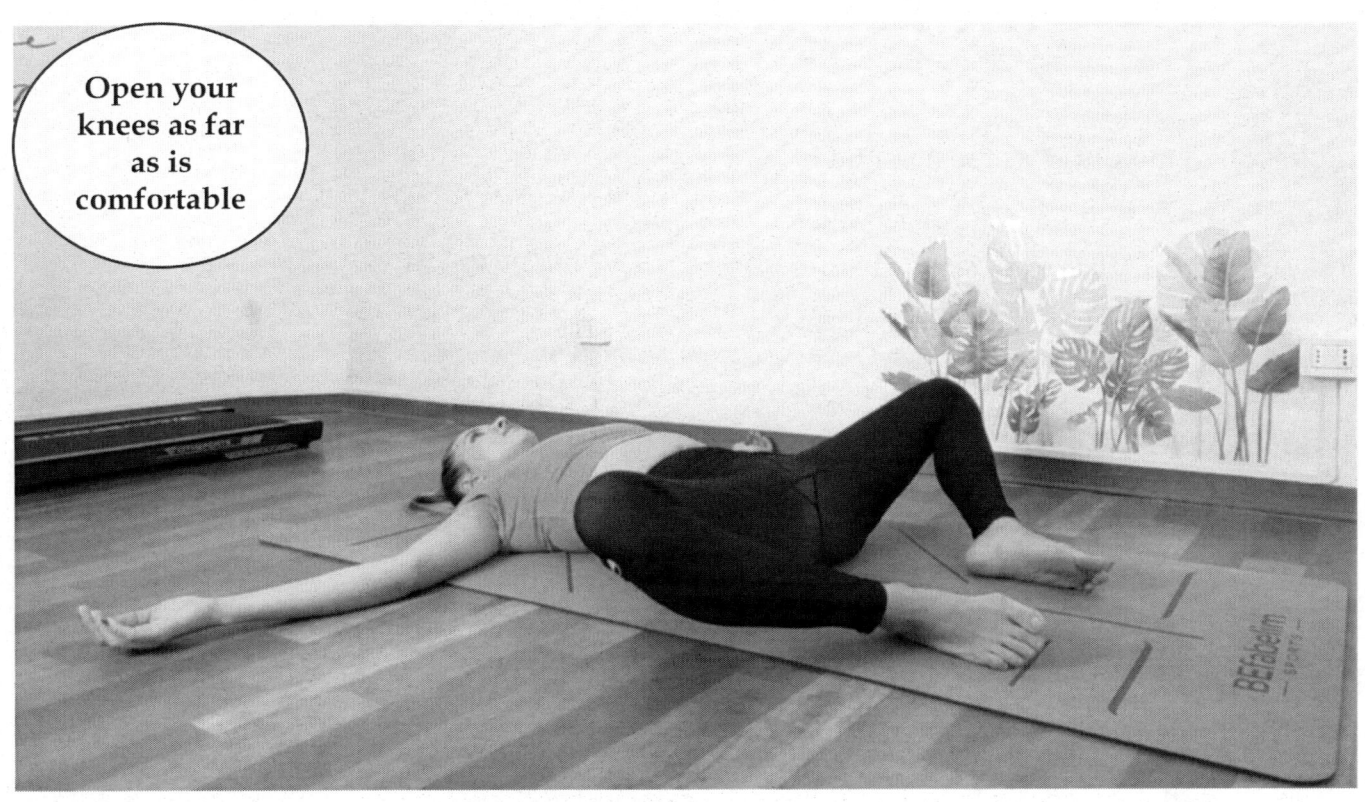

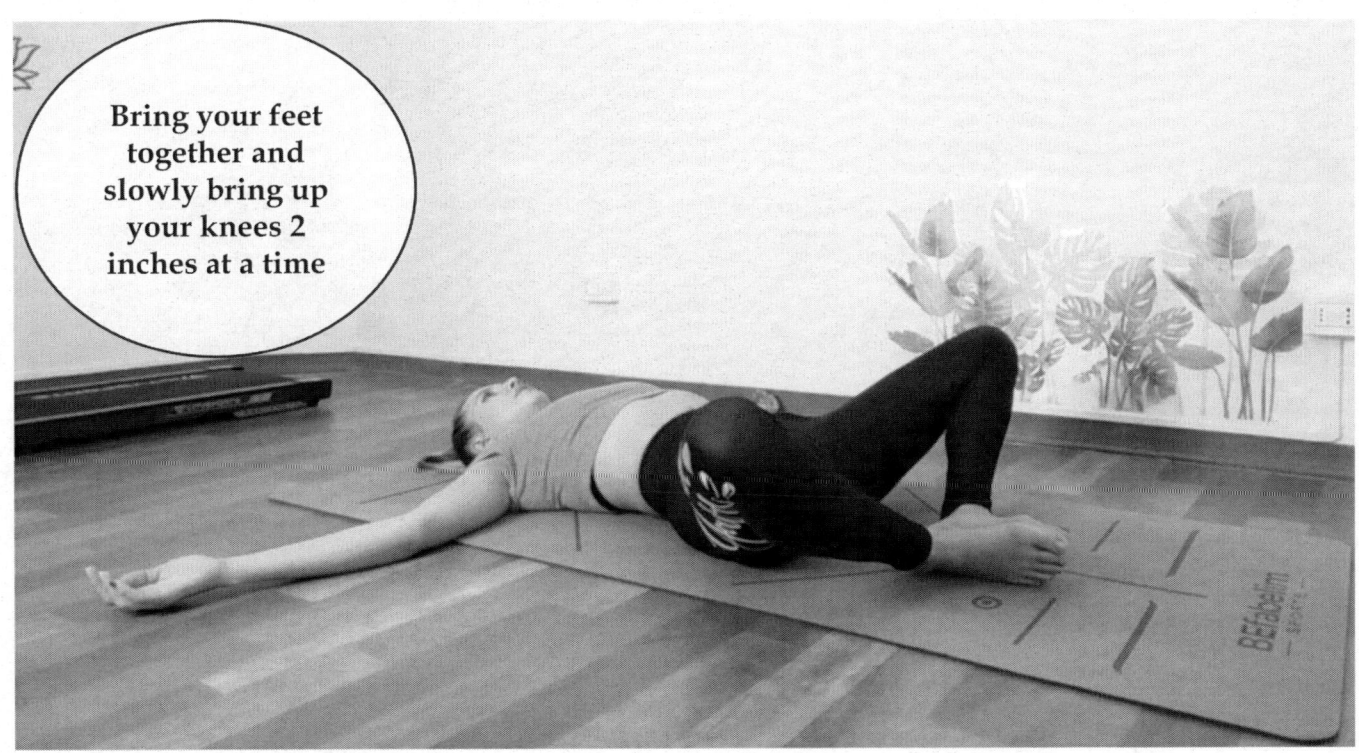

Release Trauma: Exercise 2

Benefits

Trauma often manifests as tension and holding patterns in the body. This second exercise helps to release physical tension, allowing you to let go of the physiological effects of trauma.

Instructions

1. Stand tall with your feet hip distance apart. Now very slowly lower down into a squat until your buttocks touch the ground and then completely release your back down onto the mat.

2. Take a couple of breaths and repeat the exercise.

Breathing

Inhale before the squat

Exhale during the squat.

Repetitions, Sets, and Rest

8 repetitions, resting for 10 seconds each set.

Suitable for

Trauma Release.

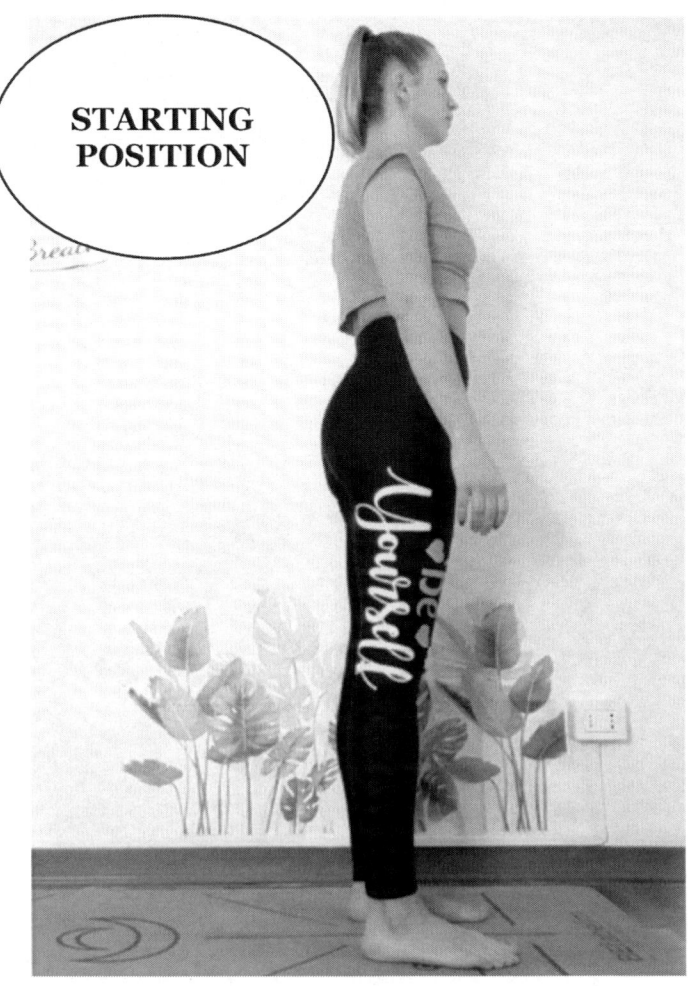

STARTING POSITION

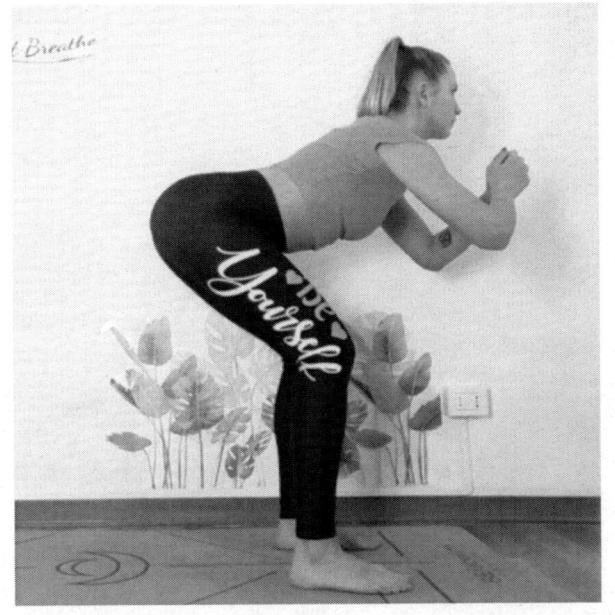 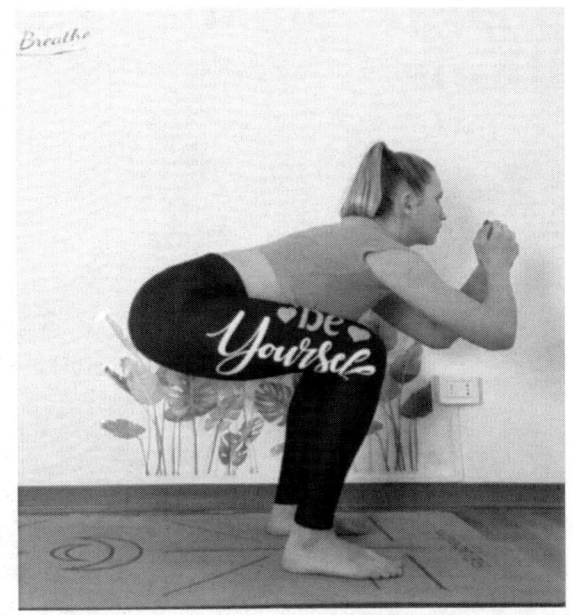

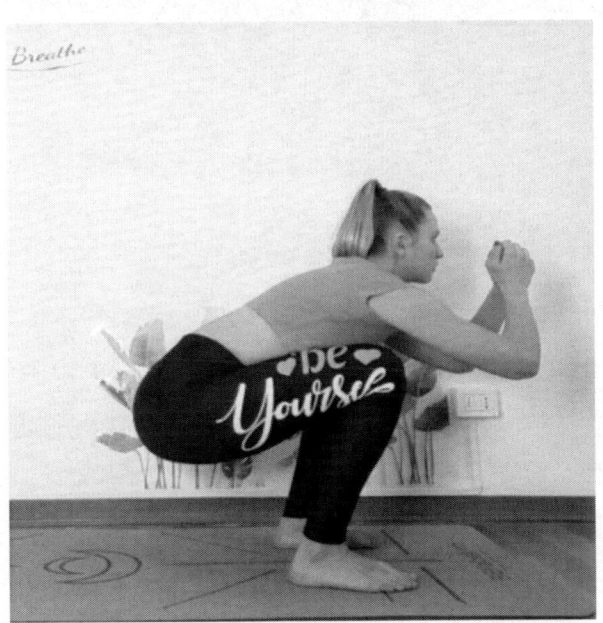 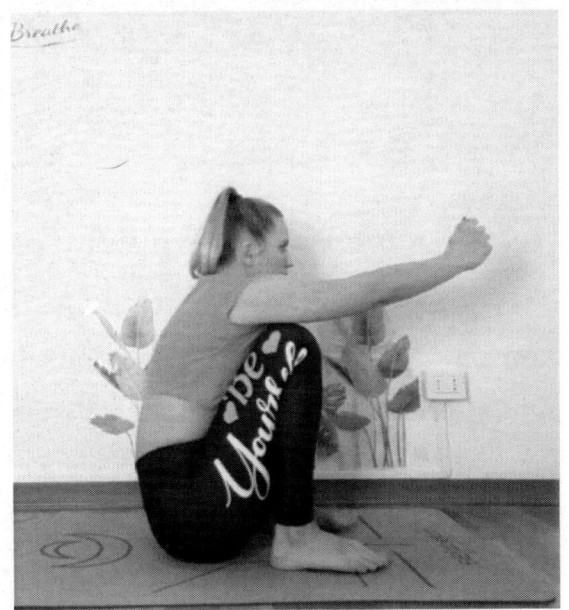

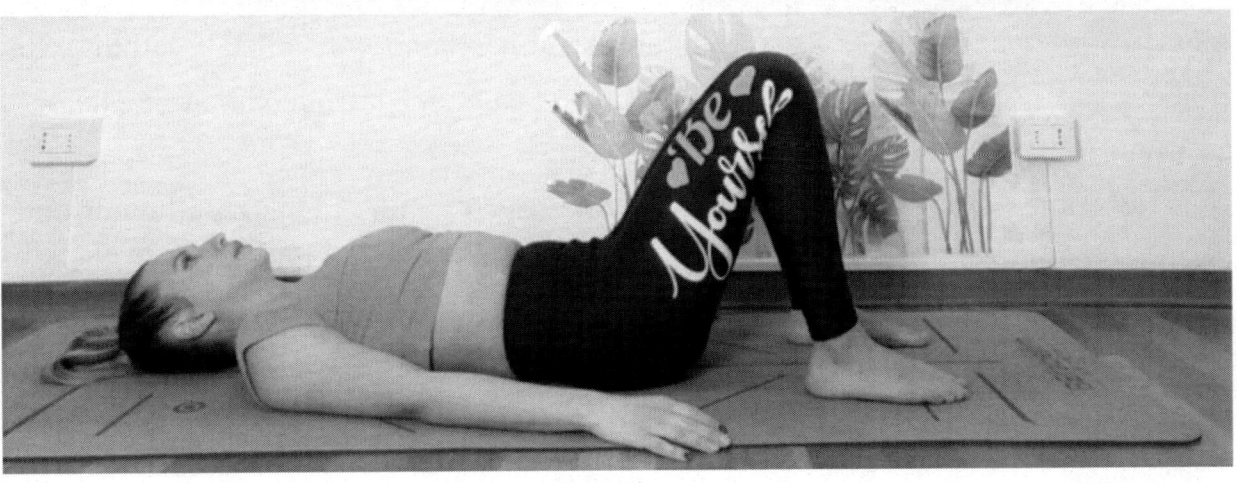

Chapter 3: Somatic Exercises for Stress Relief and Breathing

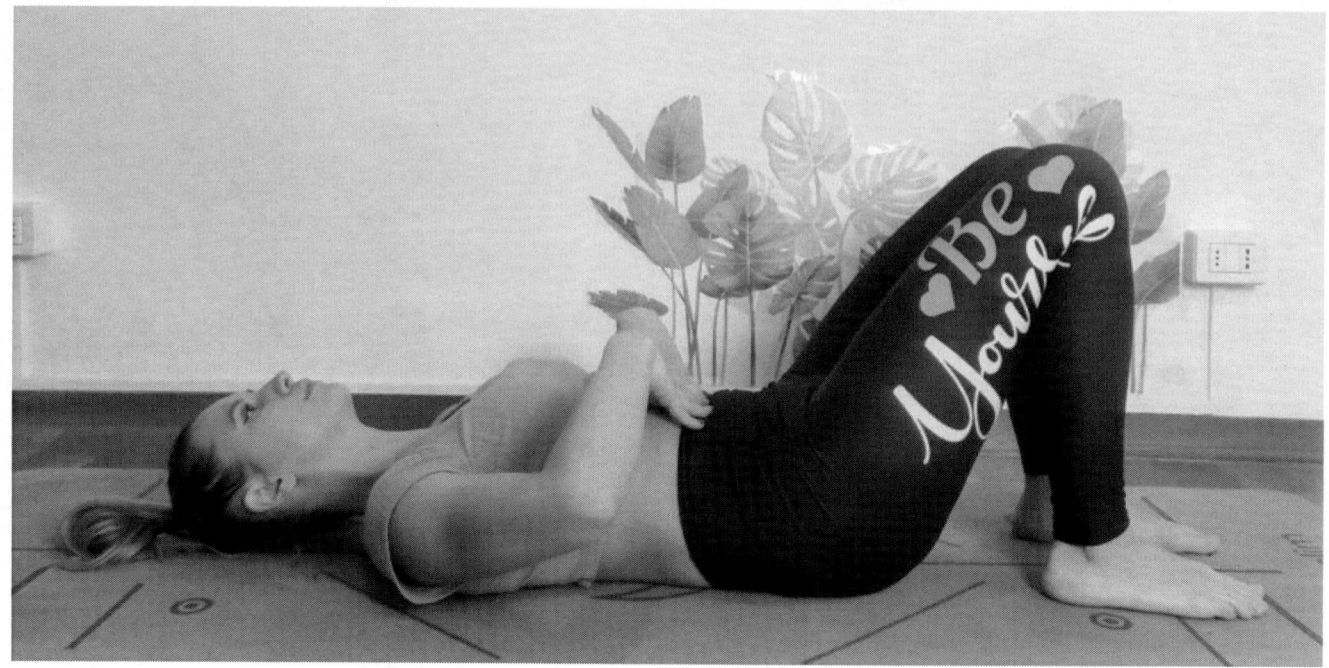

Somatic exercises may be a very useful tool for stress relief.

Somatics is a low-impact training technique that emphasizes strengthening, flexibility, and general body awareness. Controlled motions, breathing exercises, and an emphasis on posture and alignment are all part of the practice. These components may lessen stress in a number of ways:

Mind-body connection: Somatics helps to establish a strong mental-physical bond. Being more mindful of your breathing, posture, and movements may help you become more focused and present, which helps reduce stress.

Deep breathing: Somatics places a strong emphasis on regulated, controlled breathing, which soothes the nervous system. In addition to promoting relaxation, controlled breathing helps lower the production of stress chemicals.

Physical advantages: The physical facets of Somatics, such as muscular strengthening and stretching, may aid in releasing physical stress-related tension in the body. A more at ease and calm body state may also result from better posture and body awareness.

Endorphin Release: Exercise, particularly Somatics, causes endorphins to be released, which uplifts your mood organically. These "feel good" substances have the power to reduce stress and elevate your mood.

Somatics Exercises to Reduce Stress: to Try Right Now

Reducing speed in the highly connected culture of today is a difficult endeavor! We are constantly overtaken by distractions. When our focus is often drawn in multiple ways, it may be challenging to focus and have a composed attitude. Thankfully, research has shown that Somatics is among the best exercises for reducing both physical and mental stress.

Somatics is an exercise that employs body-stretching and strengthening movements to emphasize core strength and flexibility. People of many ages and backgrounds are increasingly using this strategy due to its growing popularity worldwide.

Have you ever noticed how tension and stress may negatively impact your health and increase your susceptibility to disease? Stress is known to have detrimental impacts on both our physical and mental health.

Somatics may assist in reducing the harmful consequences of stress. Practicing Somatics gives you the space to not only be conscious of the current moment but also to better handle the stresses of life by helping you to concentrate on your body, mind, and breathing. You'll get physical advantages like better posture, flexibility, and core strength, but it will also help you feel calmer and more relaxed, which will lift your spirits and make you feel better all around.

In addition, it enhances your body awareness, boosts your mood and vitality, sharpens your memory and focus, and aids in better sleep hygiene.

Five Somatics poses that effectively reduce stress.

You may enhance your general mental health and lessen the symptoms of anxiety and sadness by adding these exercises to your Somatics practice. Breathe deeply, concentrate on the motions, and release any problems or distractions. Try these exercises and see how they work for you. Somatic may be a wonderful tool for decreasing stress and increasing mental health.

Stress-relieving activities in Somatics usually include deep breathing, slow, deliberate movements, and visualization exercises.

These techniques for lowering stress may be included in your Somatics
 practice to help you de-stress and relax. You may also develop a feeling of awareness and calm that you can bring into your regular life by paying attention to your breathing and the way your body moves.

Exercises 1 – 2 for Stress Relief: Wall Roll Down / Roll UP

Benefits

Spinal flexibility. Stretching the hamstrings, back, and abdominals.

Use this exercise as a link between your Somatics routine and daily life to help you incorporate good posture. Include this exercise in your daily routine.

Instructions

1. Stand up against the wall; ensure your upper back, shoulders, and hands remain on the wall throughout the exercise.

2. Begin by slowly curling your head forward, moving one vertebra at a time.

3. When your chin touches the chest, hold this position for 10 seconds not allowing the shoulders to leave the wall.

4. Slowly and in a controlled motion, raise your head back to the starting position.

Breathing

Inhale when your chin reaches the chest.

Exhale as you back in the starting position.

Repetitions, Sets, and Rest

from 5 to 10 reps for 2 – 3 sets, resting for 20 seconds between each.

Suitable for

Improve Spinal flexibility.

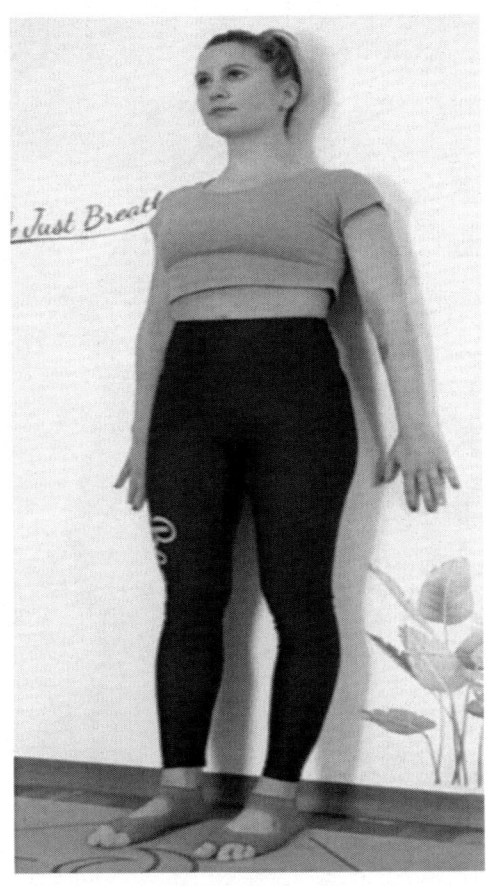

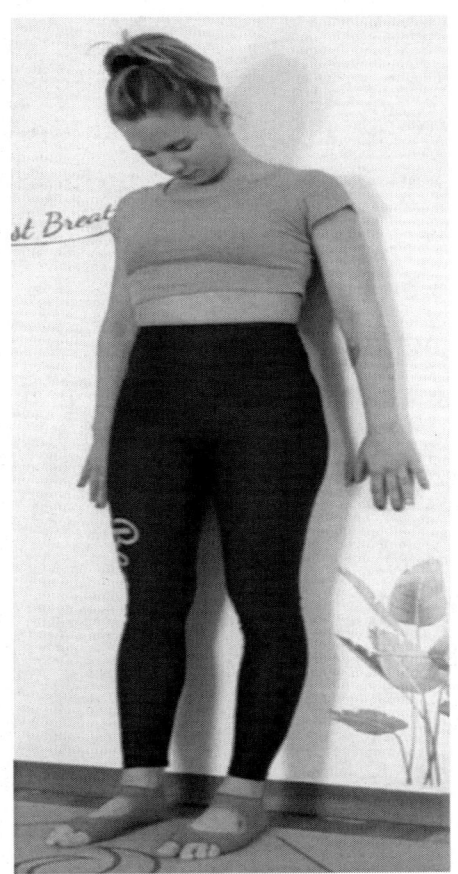

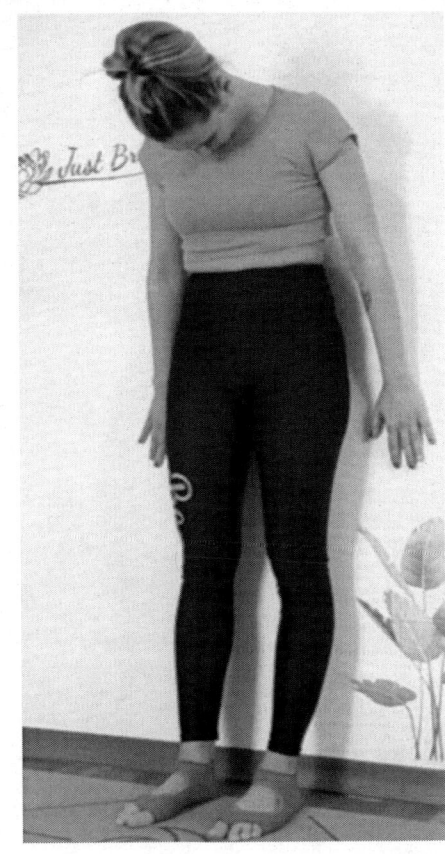

Exercise 3 for Stress Relief: Wall Angels

Benefits

This exercise provides traction, separates the vertebrae, flattens curves, and improves posture.

Instructions

1. Stand with your feet about a foot away from the wall, knees bent around 20-25 degrees.
2. Press your lower back (pelvic tilt) against the wall.
3. Lift your arms against the wall at 90 degrees and raise them off the wall.
4. Hold the position for 1-2 seconds then lower your arms at 90 degrees.

Breathing

Inhale as you raise your arms off the wall.

Exhale as you lower your arms.

Repetitions and Sets

4 – 5 arm movements for 1 set.

Suitable for

Posture improving.

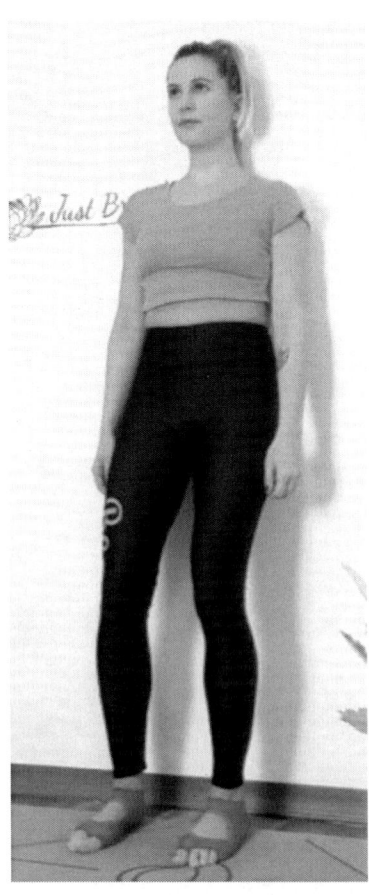
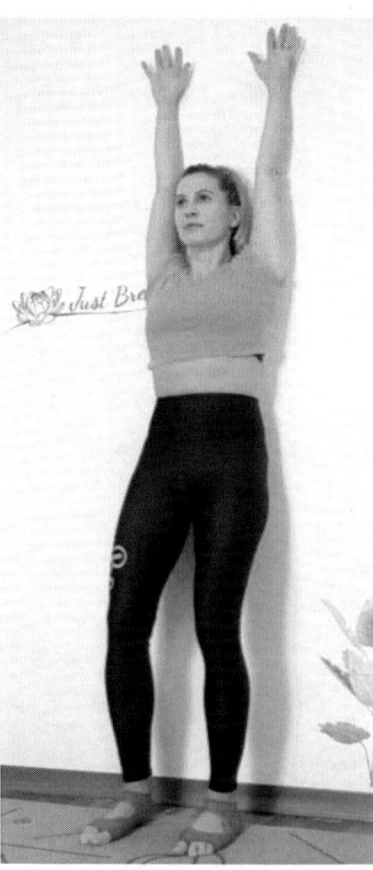
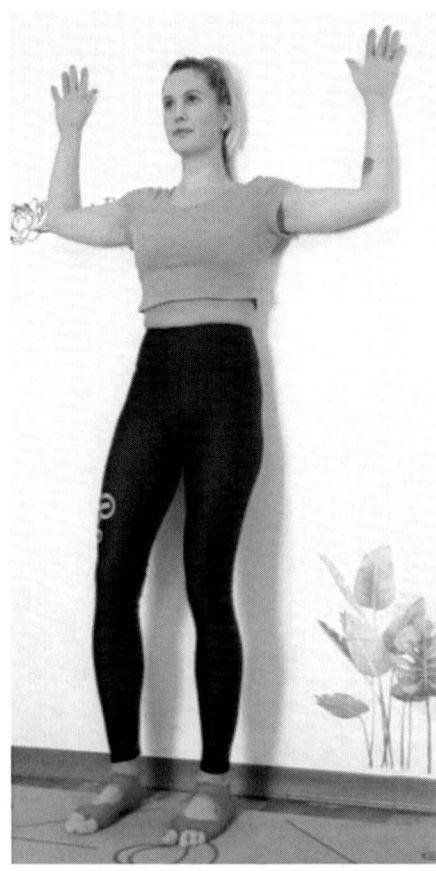

Exercise 4 for Stress Relief: Wall Tree Pose

Benefits

This exercise enhances focus and concentration, and it improves balance, stability, and flexibility.

Instructions

1. Stand in front of the wall, with your back that touches the wall to facilitate the balance.
2. Lift your right leg and place the foot onto your inner thigh.

TIP: Adjust leg placement for comfort, avoiding the inner knee.

3. Extend arms upward or in a comfortable position, focusing on balance.
4. Repeat the exercise with the other hand.

Breathing

Deeply Inhale allowing the breath to fill your lungs.

Slowly Exhale through the nose or mouth.

Repetitions and Sets

5 – 10 breaths each side.

Suitable for

Balance, stability and flexibility enhance.

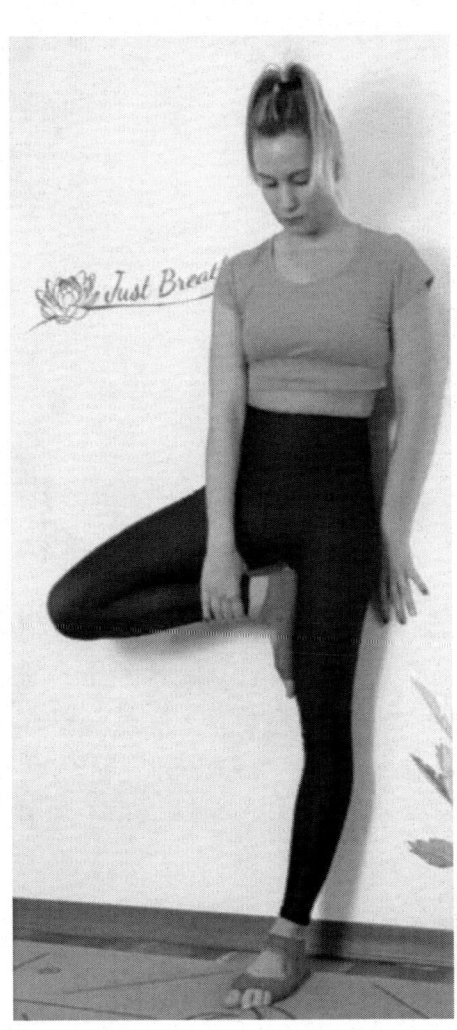
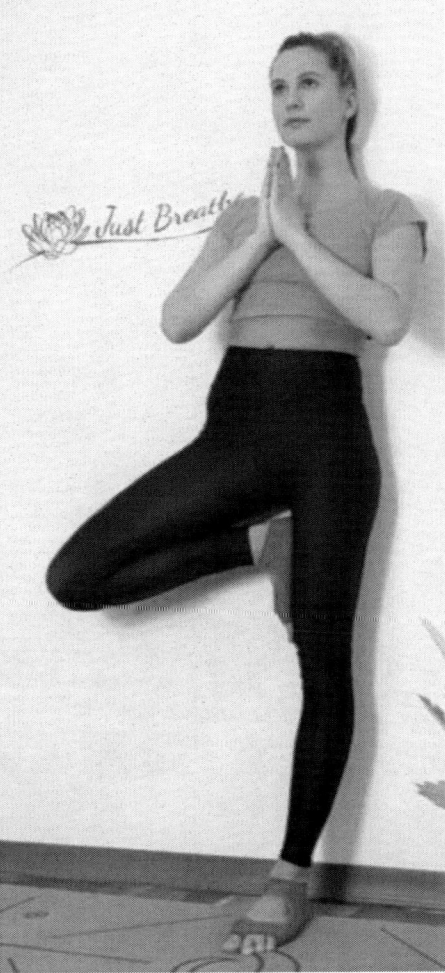
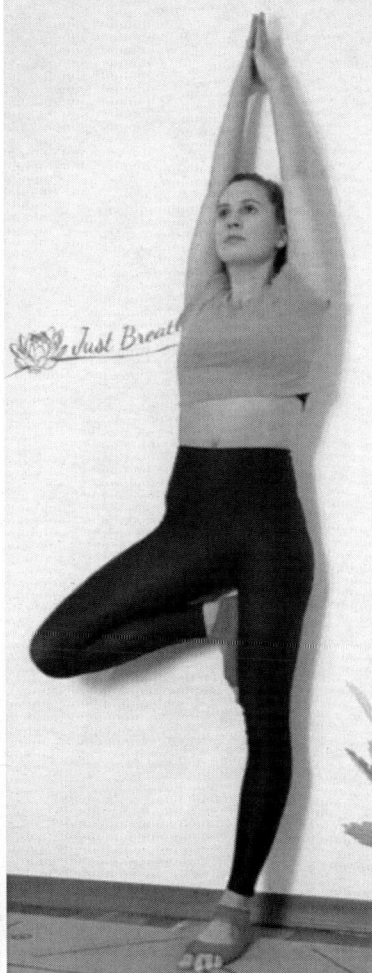

Exercise 5 for Stress Relief: Wall Butterfly

Benefits

This exercise opens up the inner thigh muscles.

Instructions

1. Lie on your back with your legs elevated against the wall, ensuring your hips are in contact with the wall.
2. Bring the soles of your feet together in front of your body and allow your knees to open to each side.
3. Hold your feet with your hands and rest your elbows on your knees.
4. open the knees/legs as far as you can.

TIP: Place your hands on your legs and gently push to increase the stretch.

5. After a few breaths, hold the position, then return to the starting position.

Breathing

Deeply Inhale allowing the breath to fill your lungs.
Slowly Exhale through the nose or mouth.

Repetitions and Sets

Hold the stretch for 30 – 60 seconds for 1 – 2 sets.

Suitable for

Stretch your inner thigh muscles.

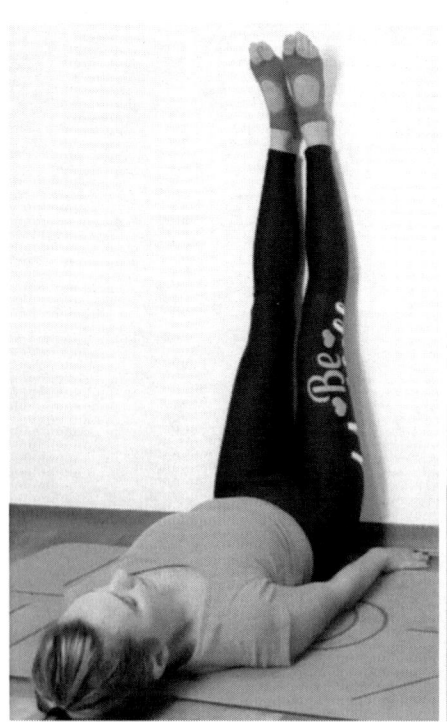 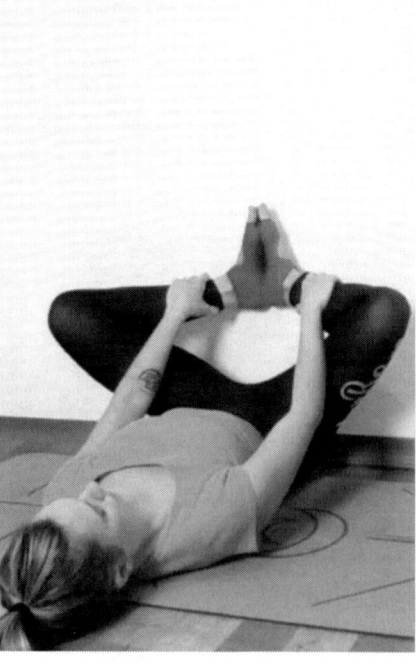 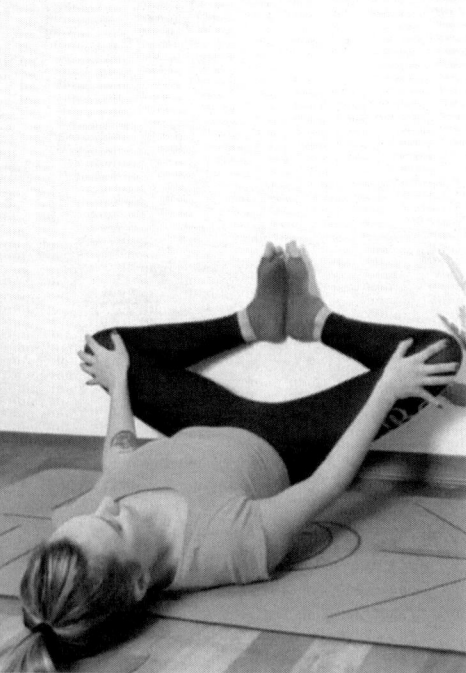

CLAIM YOUR INCLUDED BONUSES

Scan the **QR CODE** below to the **LIFETIME ACCESS** (including **download** opportunity) to the **Free Video Course, the 28-Day Plan, and all the other FREE bonuses**:

OR CLICK THE LINK BELOW:

https://drive.google.com/drive/folders/1MFSMz9 NMzlFRdLM0GoBVr7gzDAY4NpU_?usp=sharing

Please be aware that **using the QR Code does NOT require a credit card**. **Everything is completely free.**

If you are asked to use a credit card, please try a different QR code reader tool, as it might be an advertisement appearing in your current app.

If you encounter any issues, please feel free to contact me at:

aliciadiamond.fitness@gmail.com

*WAIT.. Ther's more... I have other **3 exclusive secret GIFTS** just for you!*

Are you curious to learn more? Send me an email at:

aliciadiamond.fitness@gmail.com

with the subject line:

"How to Claim my Somatics Secret Gifts"

I will get back to you within a few hours.

Chapter 4: Somatic Exercises for Stretching and Posture Perfection

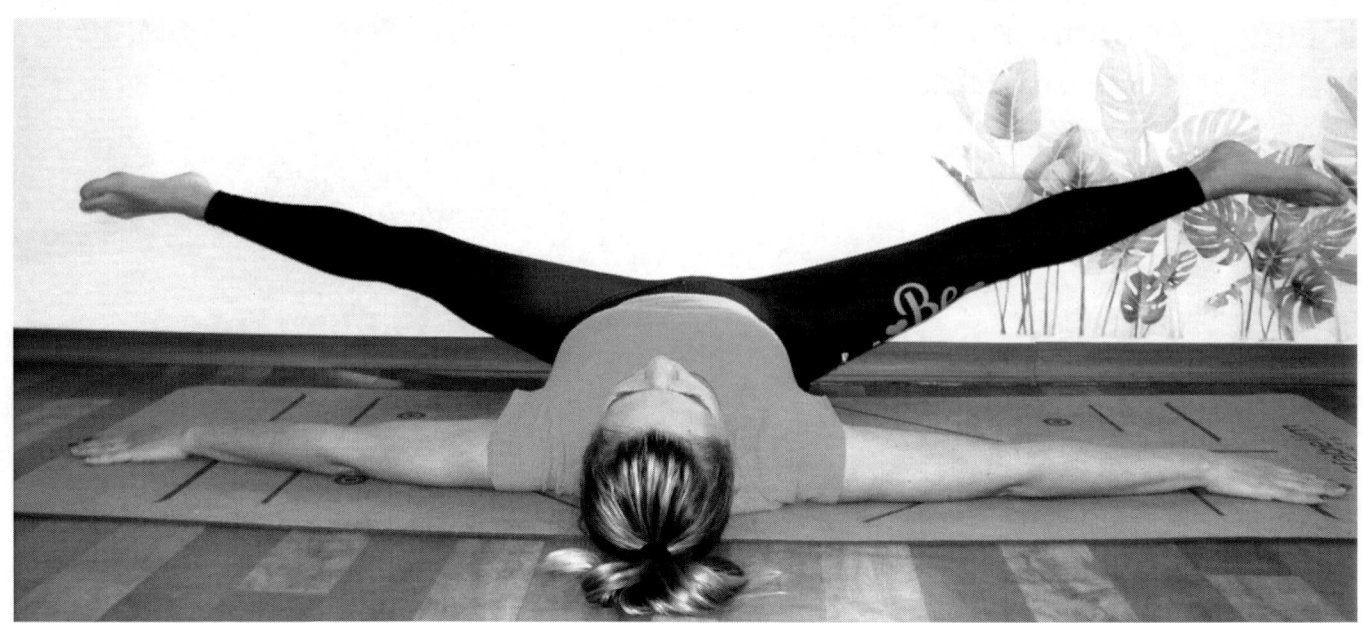

Eight Essential Guidelines:

Breathing: Using complete inhalations and exhalations, forcefully pump air into and out of the body.

Centering: Keeping your body and mind focused during each activity. Somatic exercises call the core region the "powerhouse", which is located between the ribs and hips.

Concentration: Give each exercise mor

e weight and form than repetitions. Being inwardly focused and paying great attention to the intricacies of each exercise is essential.

Control: Always stressing total bodily control while being aware of how the various components move in unison.

Flow: Stressing unbroken motion that transitions smoothly from one exercise to the next without sacrificing style.

Precision: Follow the instructions step-by-step and execute each exercise precisely. moves.

Core engagement: The core serves as the central support of the body, comprising not only superficial muscles but also deeper stabilizing components.

Pelvic Floor: the pelvic floor emerges as an often overlooked yet integral element. This network of muscles and connective tissue beneath the pelvis serves multifaceted purposes, supporting organs, maintaining continence, and contributing significantly to core stability.

CORE Engagement: The Dying Bug

Benefits

It's essential to activate the pelvic floor and engage the core.

Core Strengthening targets the transverse abdominis, contributing to core strength and stability, which is crucial for posture and overall body strength.

This exercise strengthens the core, improves coordination, and enhances flexibility.

Instructions

1. While lying flat on your back, raise your arms straight up toward the ceiling and place your legs in a tabletop posture.
2. Flat your right leg and left arm towards the floor.
3. Hold the position for few seconds then return to the starting position.
4. Perform the exercise with the opposite leg and arm.

Breathing

Inhale before flatting your legs and arms. Exhale when you return in the starting position.

Repetitions, Sets, and Rest

Perform 8 reps each side for 1 to 2 sets, resting for 30 to 60 seconds between each set.

Suitable for

Activate the pelvic floor and engage the core.

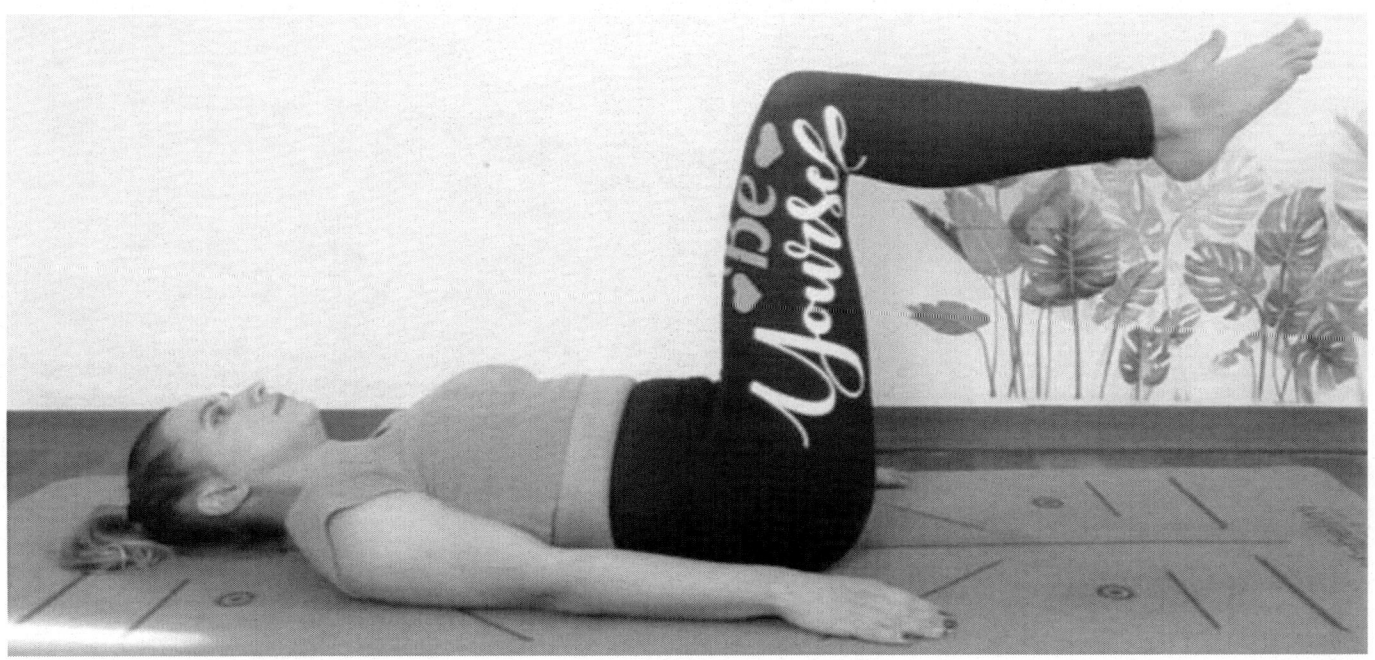

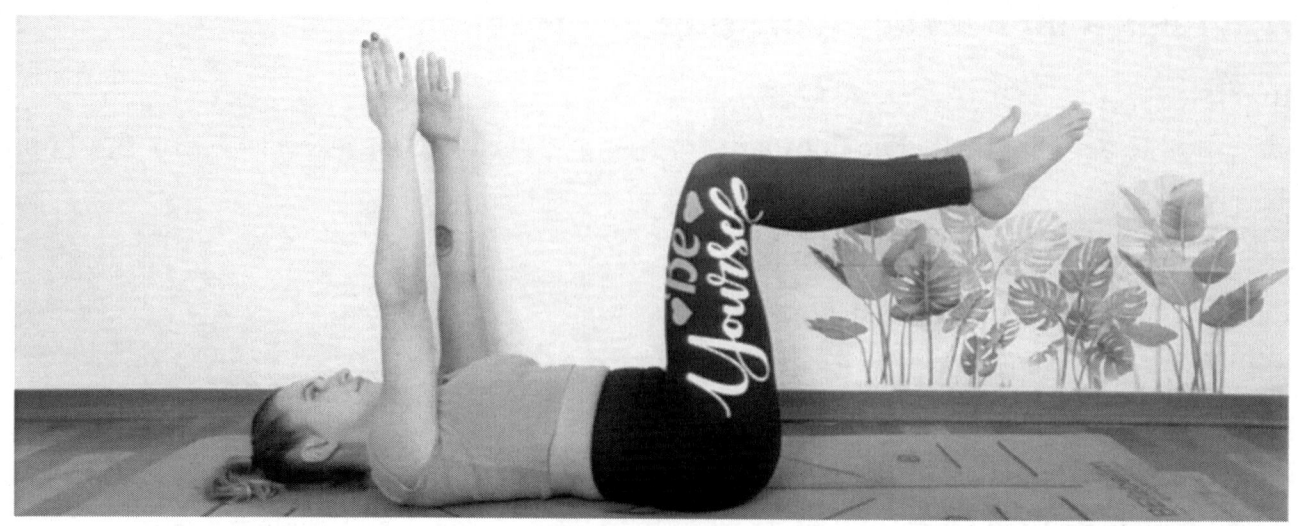

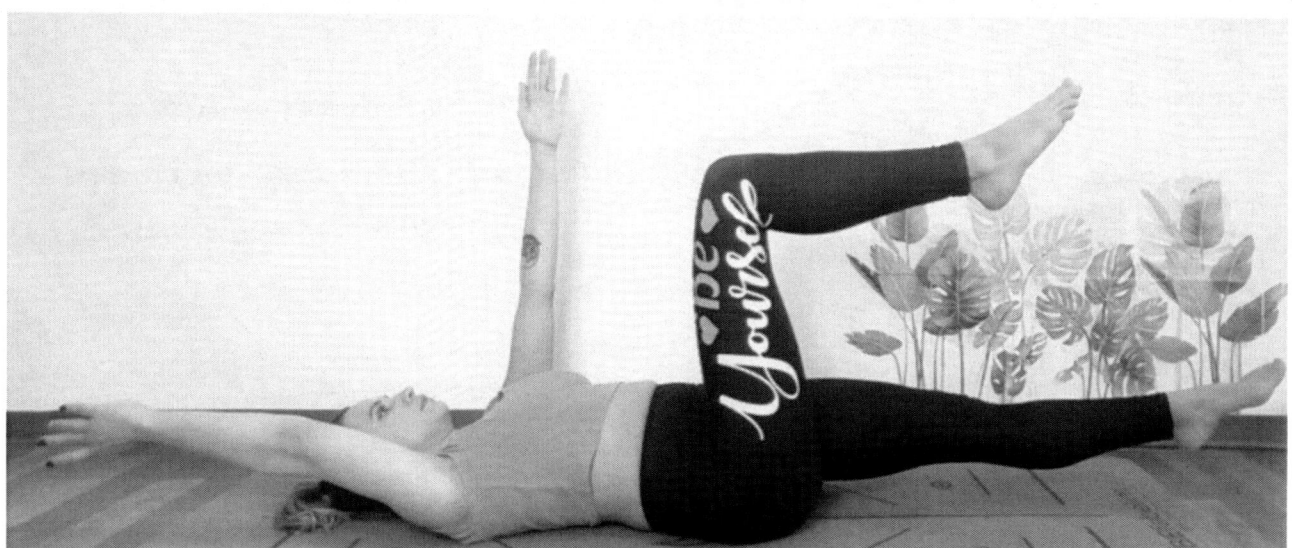

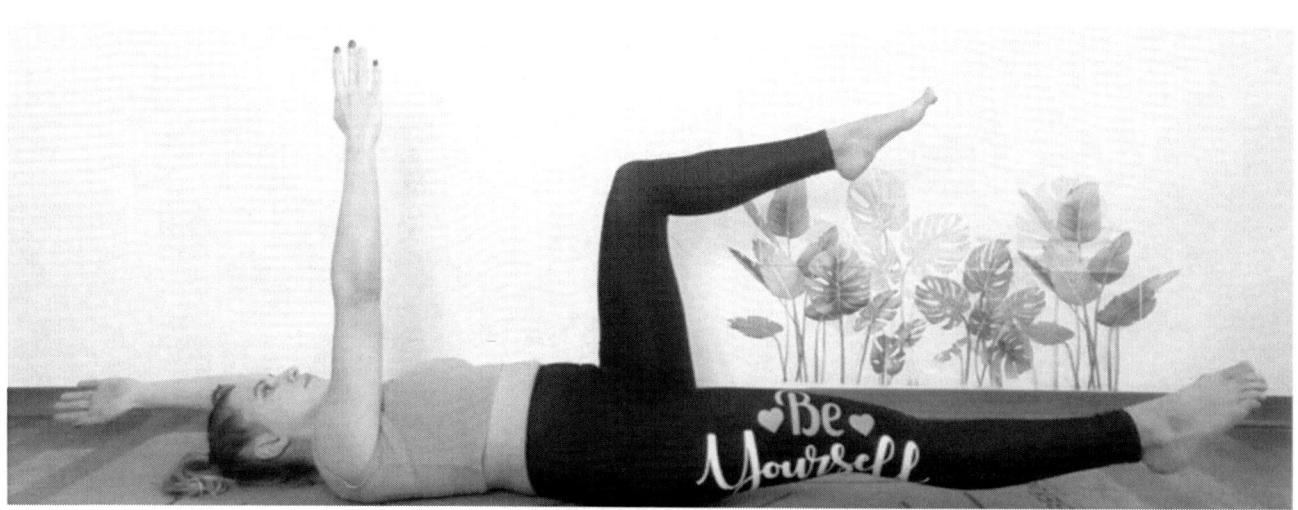

Pelvic Floor Activation

Benefits

Activating the pelvic floor muscles is beneficial for maintaining pelvic health, supporting organs, and preventing issues like incontinence. Consistent practice over time can strengthen these muscles, contributing to better control and support for various bodily functions.

Instructions

1. Lie down comfortably, ensuring your body is relaxed.
2. Imagine trying to stop the flow of urine or prevent passing gas, and tighten the pelvic floor muscles as if performing those actions. Avoid excessive tightening of the abdomen, buttocks, or legs.
3. Hold the contraction for about 3-5 seconds, maintaining a steady breath. Gradually release the muscles and relax for the same duration.

Breathing

Inhale while contracting the pelvic floor.

Exhale while releasing the pelvic floor.

Repetitions, Sets, and Rest

Perform 8–10 reps, increasing the duration of each contraction up to 10 seconds, and the number of repetitions as you become more comfortable. Aim for 1–2 sets, resting 20–30 seconds between each set.

Suitable for

Activate the pelvic floor muscles.

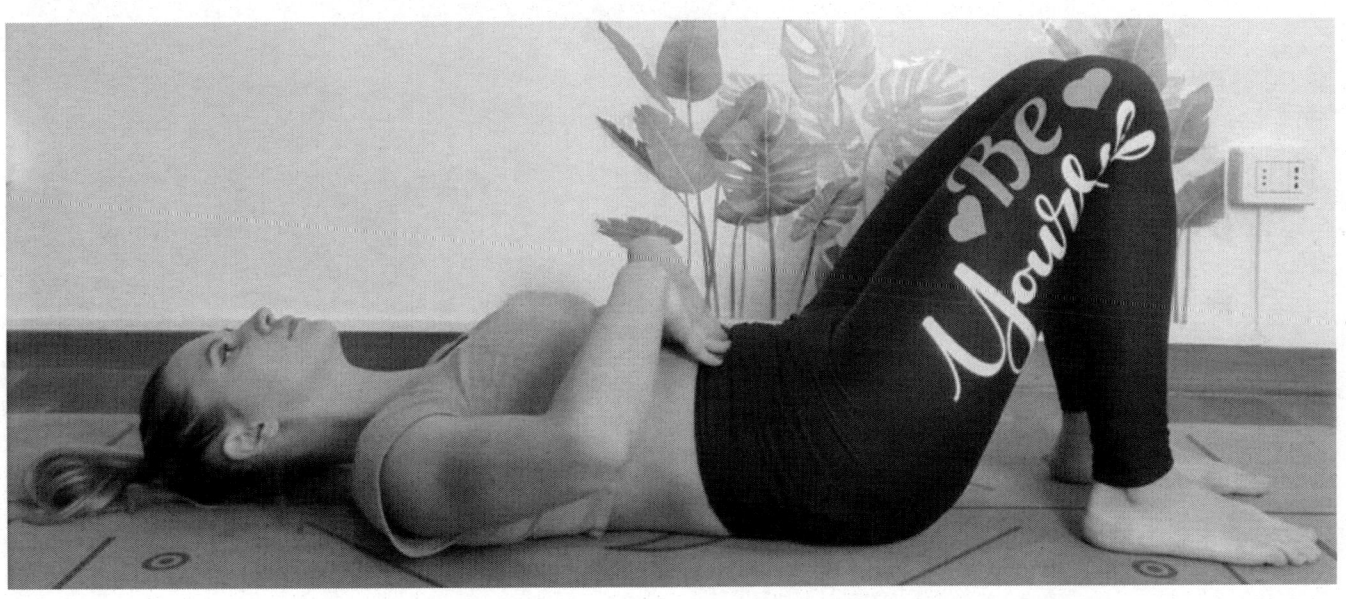

Spinal – Hamstring – Glutes: Enabled Roll Down

Benefits

This exercise helps alleviate backaches and shoulder aches, strengthens the abdominal muscles, provides a stretch for the back of the legs, and improves overall body mobility and flexibility.

Instructions

1. Sit with your feet against the wall, ensuring they remain on the floor throughout the exercise.

2. Lean your back towards your thighs while keeping your feet against the wall, maintaining contact with the floor.

3. Return to the starting position.

Breathing

Inhale as you raise yourself back to the starting position.

Exhale as you reach the bottom of the roll.

Repetitions, Sets, and Rest

10 repetitions for 1 – 2 sets, resting for 30 – 60 seconds between each set.

Suitable for

alleviate backaches and shoulder aches.

TIPS

To ease the exercise, slightly lift your knees from the floor.

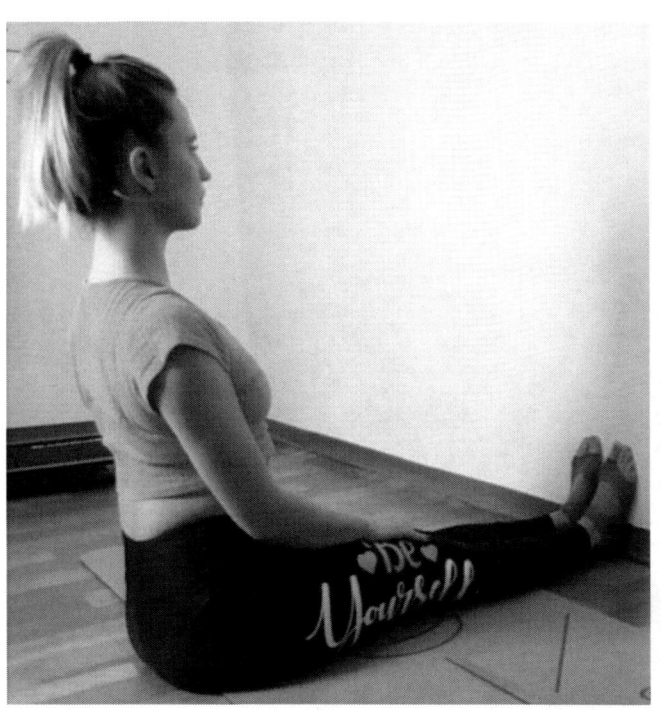 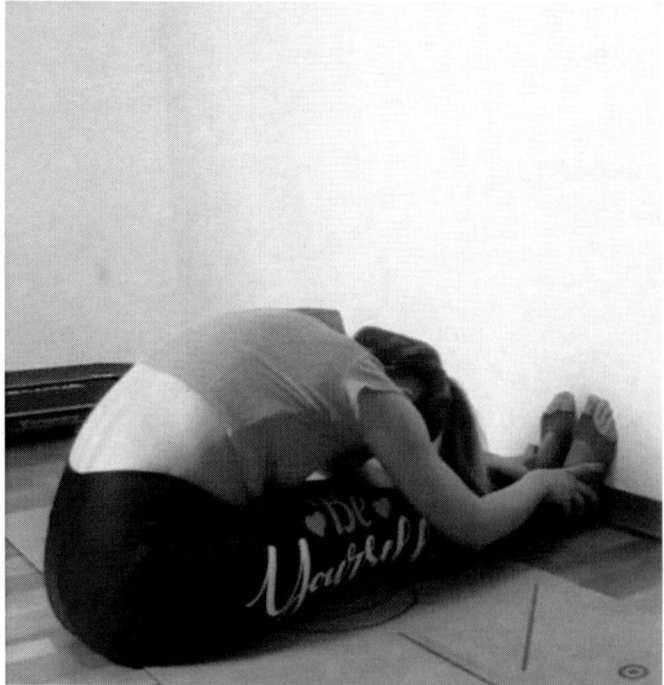

Neck Stretch

Benefits

This exercise helps to improve flexibility and mobility.

Instructions

1. Standing with your back facing the wall, put your right arm across the lower back as much as you can.
2. Hook your head with your left hand.
3. Pull your left year towards the shoulder until you feel a deep stretch.
4. Hold this position for 20 seconds.
5. Go back to the starting position and Switch sides.

Breathing

Inhale before twisting your neck.

Exhale as you twist.

Repetitions, Sets, and Rest

Hold the neck position for 20 seconds each side for 1 – 2 sets, resting for 30 seconds between each set.

Suitable for

Improve neck flexibility and mobility.

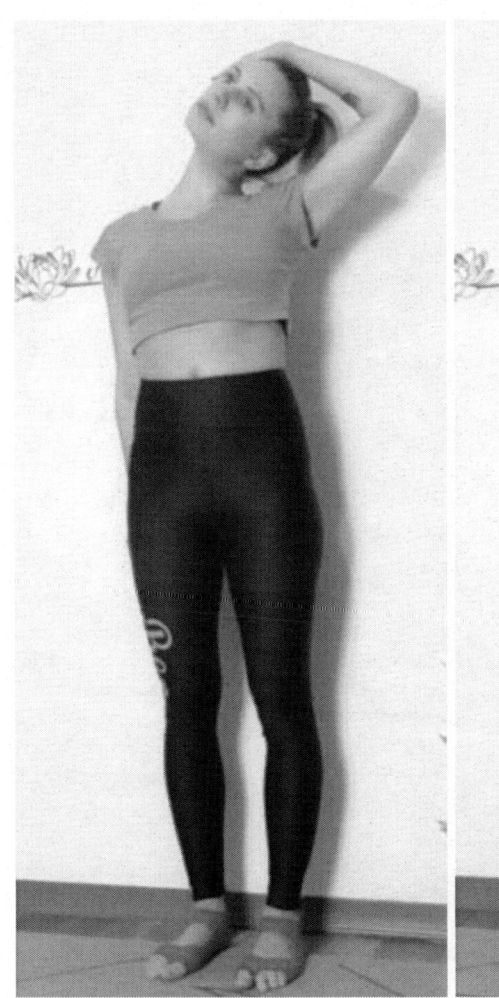
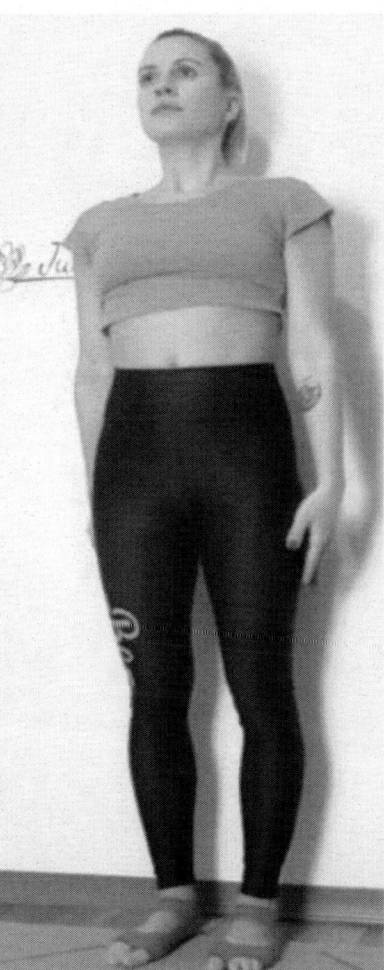
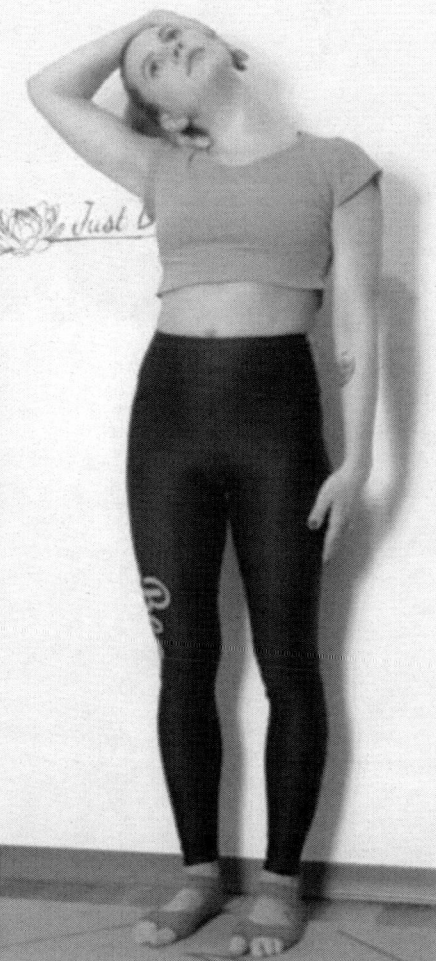

Chest Stretch

Benefits

This exercise opens up your chest and loosens your biceps and the muscles of your shoulders. It also increases your flexibility.

Instructions

1. Stand in the corner of the wall and place your palms facing the wall, positioning each hand and forearm on either side of the corner with the elbows slightly above shoulder height.

2. Slowly lean inward and bring your head and trunk as one segment toward the corner until you feel a mild stretch in your chest.

3. Hold the stretch for 20-30 seconds. In the stretched position, you can increase the stretch by squeezing your shoulder blades together.

Breathing

Deeply Inhale and Exhale during the stretch.

Repetitions, Sets, and Rest

Hold the Chest position for 30 seconds for 1 – 2 sets, resting for 30 – 60 seconds between each set.

Suitable for

Increase chest and shoulders flexibility.

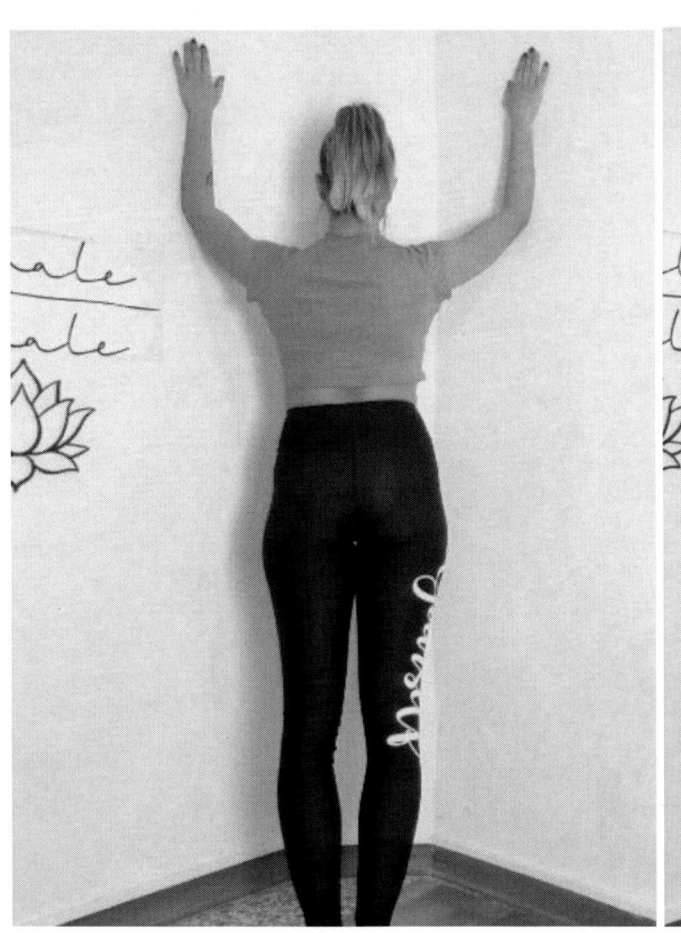 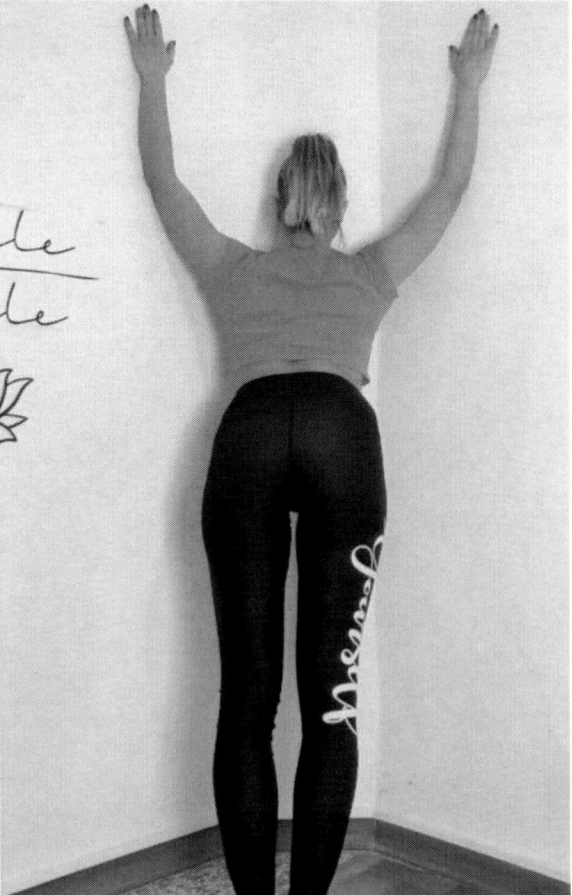

Glutes Stretch

Benefits

This exercise relieves muscle tightness and tension, reduce low back pain or tightness in your hips, increase your flexibility and range of motion.

Instructions

1. Lean the back against the Wall.
2. Raise your right knee toward your chest and cross your right foot on the left leg.
3. Hold the knee to your chest with the left hand and keep the position for 20 seconds.

4. Return to your starting posture and repeat on the opposite side of your body.

Breathing

Deeply Inhale and Exhale during the stretch.

Repetitions, Sets, and Rest

Hold the stretch position for 20 seconds for 1 – 2 sets, resting for 30 – 60 seconds between each set.

Suitable for

Relieve tightness and tension in glute muscles.

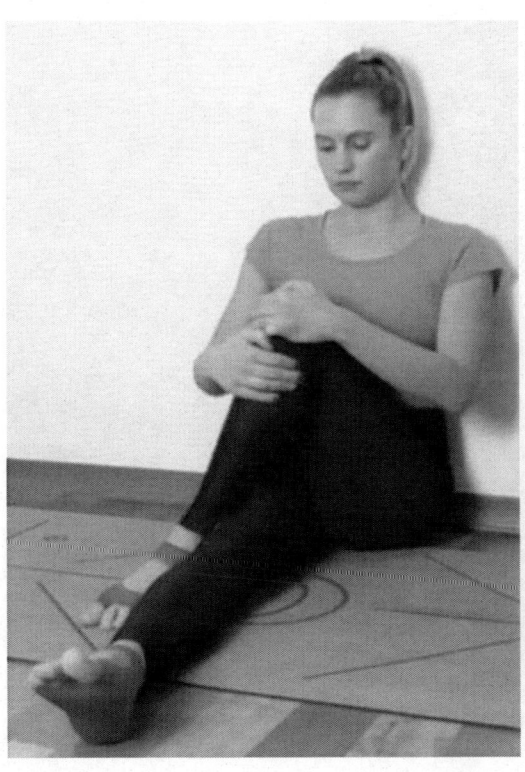
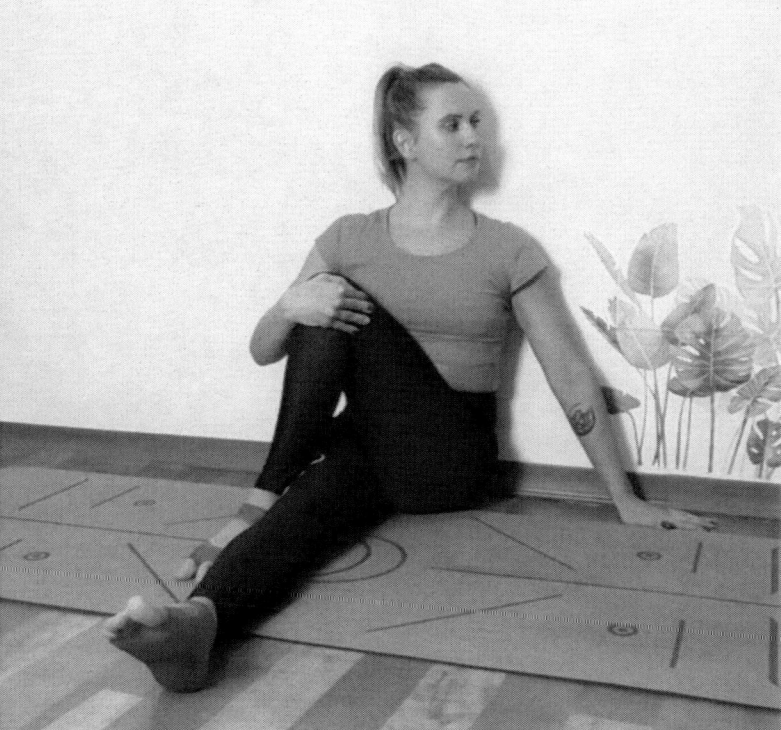

Chapter 5: Somatic Yoga Exercises A Holistic Full Body Approach

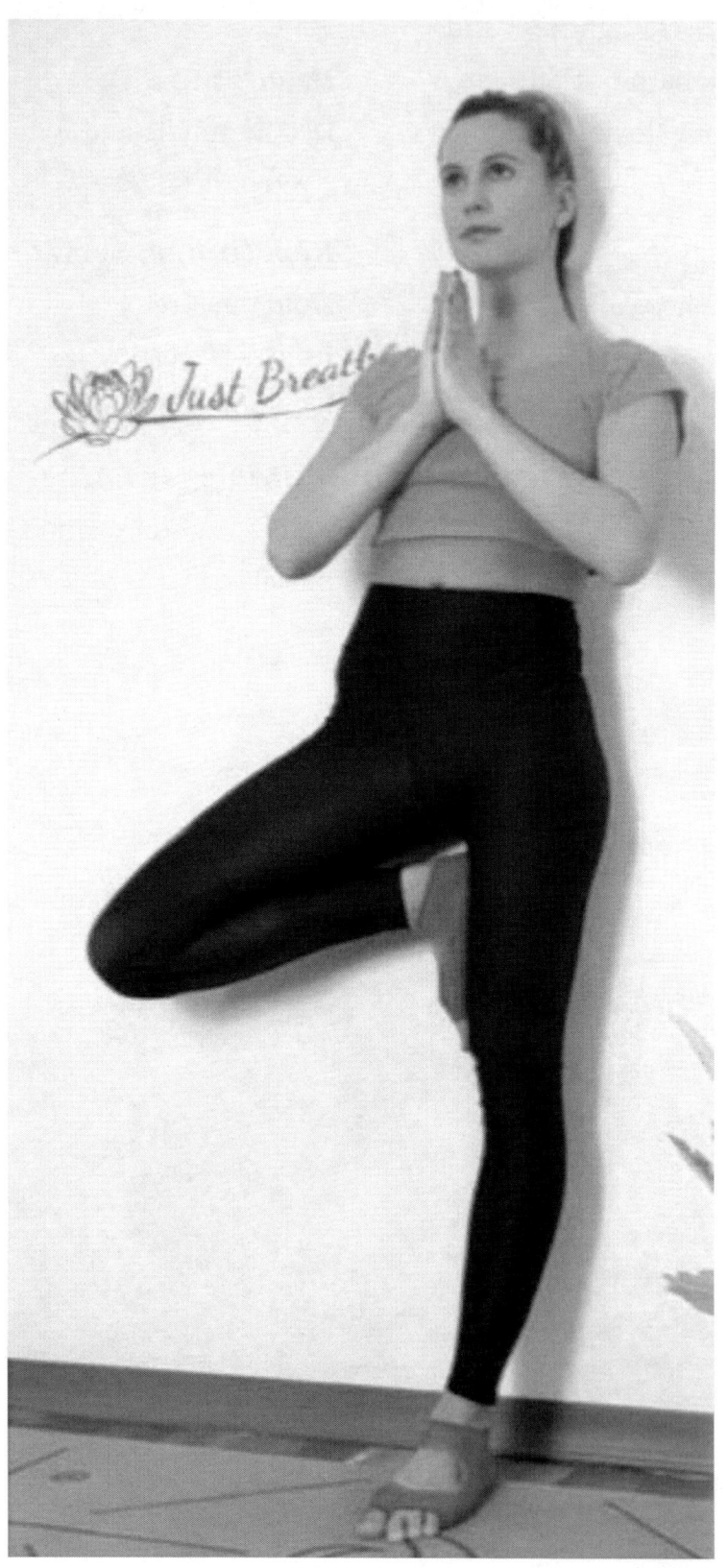

Pandiculation

Meaning

Pandiculation is a natural, instinctive movement pattern observed in animals and humans, often seen when they stretch and yawn upon waking up. This action, which involves the tightening or contracting, stretching, and then relaxing of muscles, offers several benefits, especially when consciously incorporated into one's routine through practices such as Hanna Somatic Education or certain yoga stretches. Here are some of the key benefits of pandiculation:

1. **Reduces Muscle Tension**: Pandiculation helps to reset the muscle length and reduce chronic muscle tension by signaling the nervous system to release and lengthen the muscles after they have been consciously contracted.

2. **Improves Muscle Control**: By consciously tightening and then slowly releasing muscles, you can improve your brain's control over muscle relaxation and contraction, enhancing motor control.

3. **Increases Flexibility**: Unlike passive stretching, pandiculation improves flexibility through active muscle engagement, helping to safely increase the range of motion.

4. **Relieves Stress**: The act of pandiculating can help to release physical and emotional tension, promoting relaxation and stress relief.

5. **Enhances Body Awareness**: Regularly practicing pandiculation increases proprioception, or the sense of the relative position of one's body parts, which is crucial for coordination and movement efficiency.

6. **Improves Circulation**: The process of contracting and relaxing muscles can help to stimulate blood flow, improving circulation throughout the body.

7. **Reduces Pain**: By releasing muscle tension and improving flexibility and circulation, pandiculation can help to alleviate pain, especially in cases of chronic muscle pain or stiffness.

8. **Boosts Energy**: This natural stretching and yawning process can help to wake up the body and mind, making you feel more energized and ready to start the day.

9. **Promotes Better Sleep**: Pandiculating before bed can help to relieve tension and promote relaxation, contributing to better sleep quality.

10. **Facilitates Efficient Movement**: By improving muscle control, flexibility, and body awareness, pandiculation can lead to more efficient, graceful, and effortless movement in daily life.

Pandiculation: Exercise 1 for Shoulders and Neck

Benefits

First proposed exercise to release the accumulated stress and tension in the shoulders and neck.

Instructions

1. Stand with your feet hip -width apart and bring awareness into your left shoulder.

2. Now pull your shoulder back a little bit.

3. Bring up your wrist and use your rotator cuff muscles to pull back your wrist, elbow and shoulder.

TIP: Make sure your chest is open and your head should follow the arm.

4. Hold for few seconds then release the position.

Breathing

Inhale while pulling your shoulder back.

5. Exhale to go back to the starting position.

Repetitions, Sets, and Rest

8 repetitions for 1 – 2 sets each arm, resting for 30 seconds between each set.

Suitable for

Relieve stress and tension in the shoulders and neck.

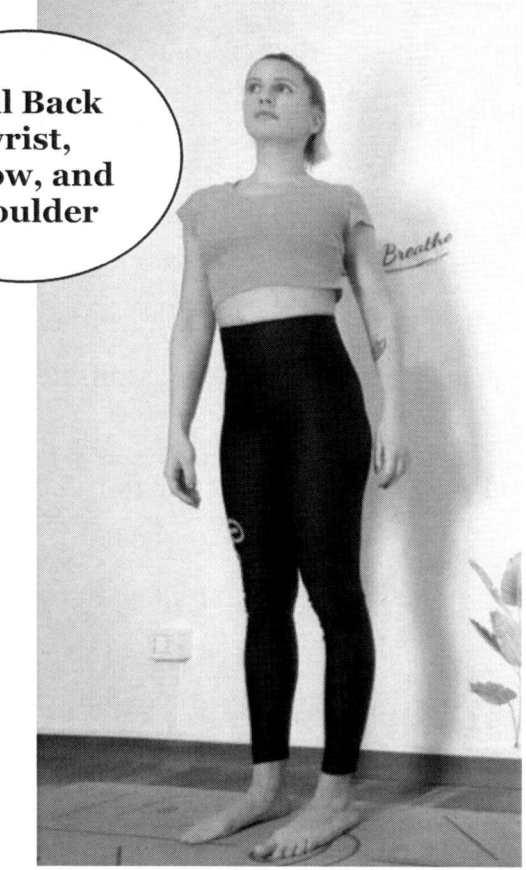

Pull Back wrist, elbow, and shoulder

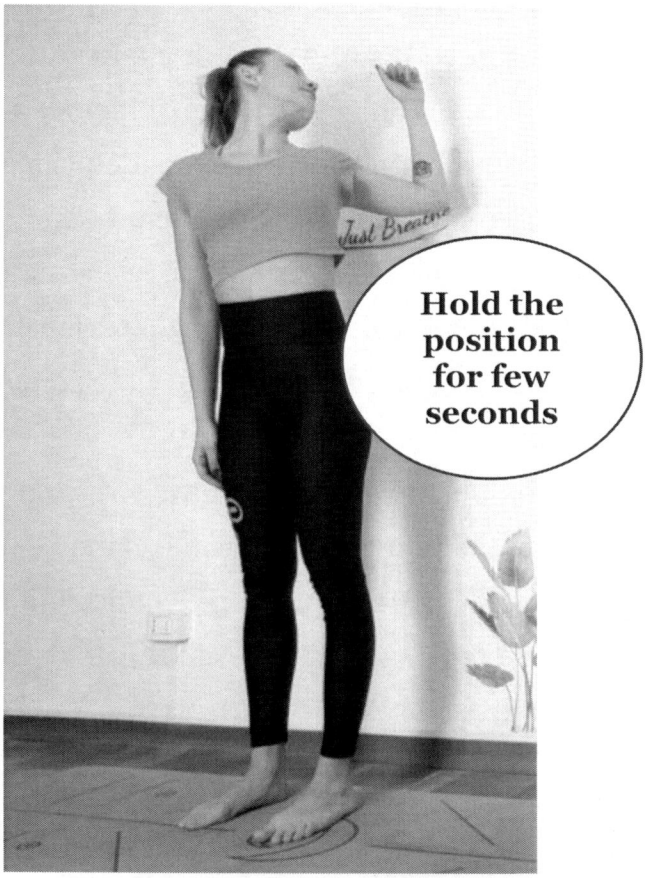

Hold the position for few seconds

Pandiculation: Exercise 2 for Shoulder and Neck

Benefits

Second proposed exercise to release the accumulated stress and tension in the shoulders and neck.

Instructions

1. Stand with your feet hip-width apart.

2. Extend your arms at chest level, palms facing down.

3. Curve your spine and move your chest away from your thumbs.

4. Hold this position for a few breaths,

5. Go back to the starting position.

Breathing

Inhale before starting the exercise.
Exhale as you push your chest against the wall.

Repetitions, Sets, and Rest

Rep from 30 to 60 seconds for 2 – 3 sets, resting for 30 seconds between each.

Suitable for

Relieve stress and tension in the shoulders and neck.

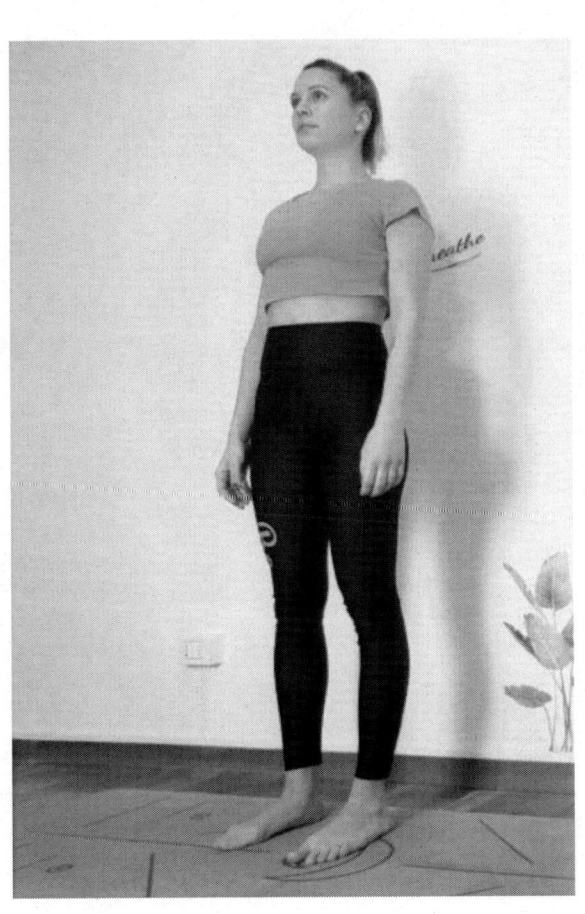

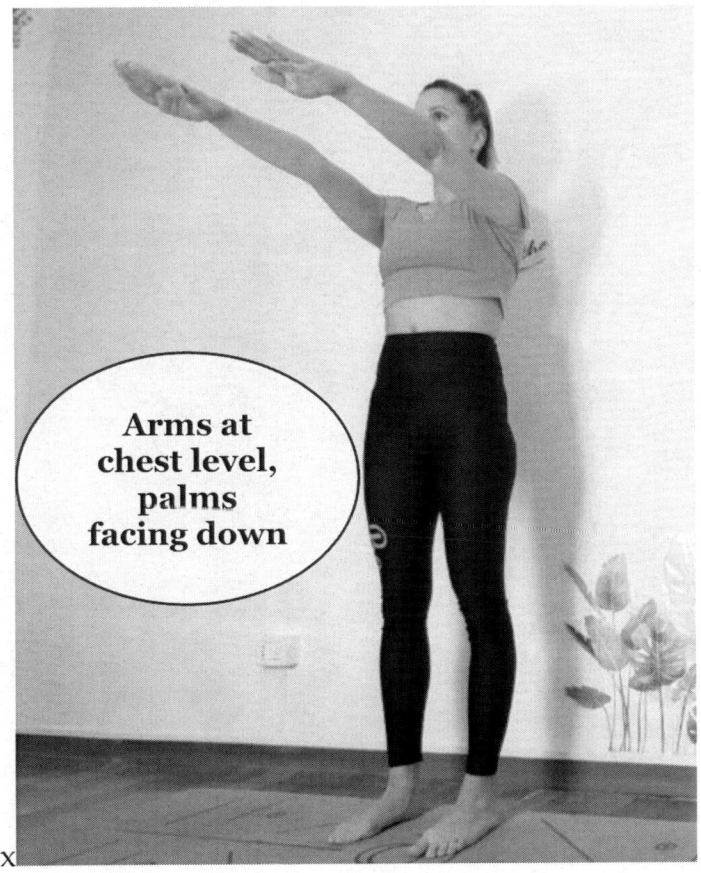

Arms at chest level, palms facing down

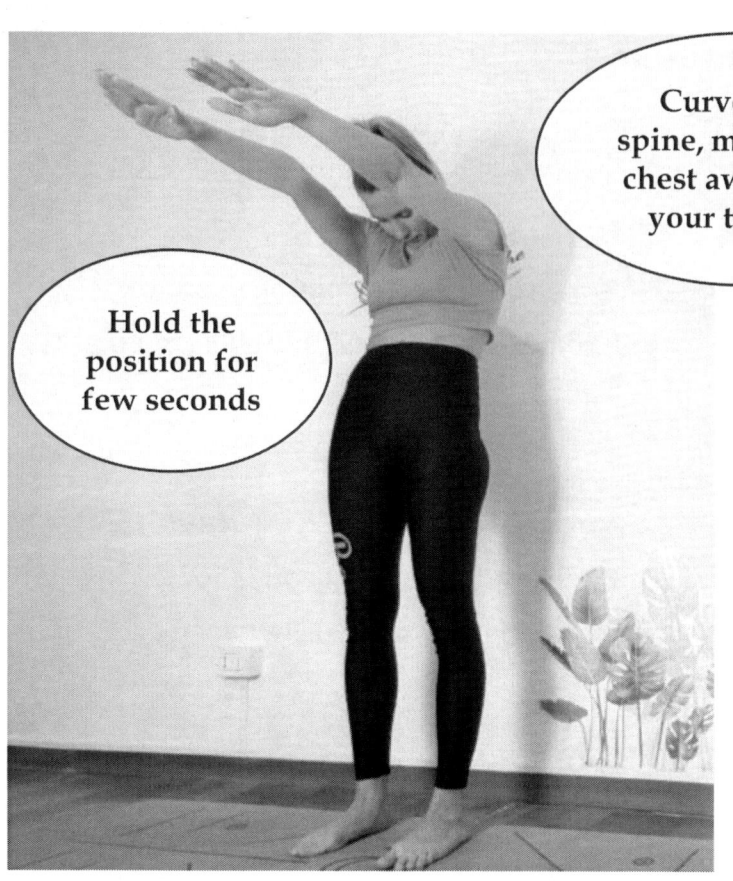

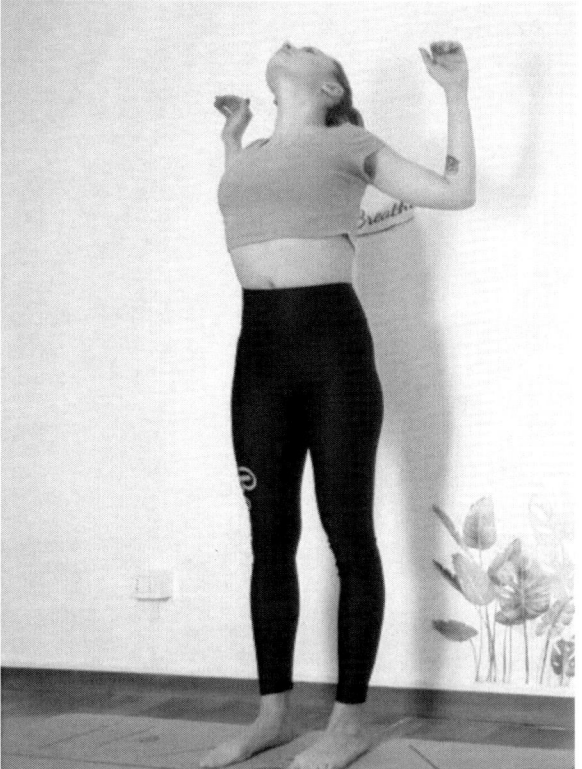

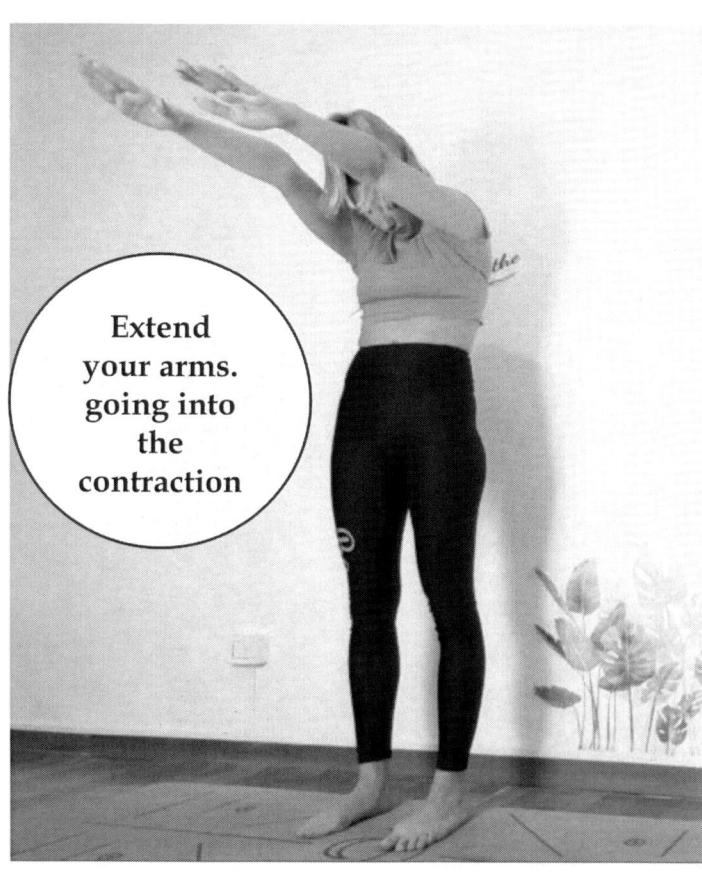

Pandiculation: Exercise 3 for Shoulder and Neck

Benefits

Third proposed exercise to release the accumulated stress and tension in the shoulders and neck.

.

Instructions

1. Stand with your feet hip -width apart.

2. Extend your right arm up

3. Slowly with your left arm try to reach the outside of your knee.

TIP: Feel the stretch in your right-side body. Keep your chest open and don't hunch your back.

4. Hold the position for few seconds then go back to the starting position and repeat on the opposite side.

5. Back to the starting position.

Breathing

Inhale while stretching to the side.

Exhale to go back to starting position.

Repetitions, Sets, and Rest

10 repetitions for 1 – 2 sets, resting for 30 seconds between each set.

Suitable for

Relieve stress and tension in the shoulders and neck.

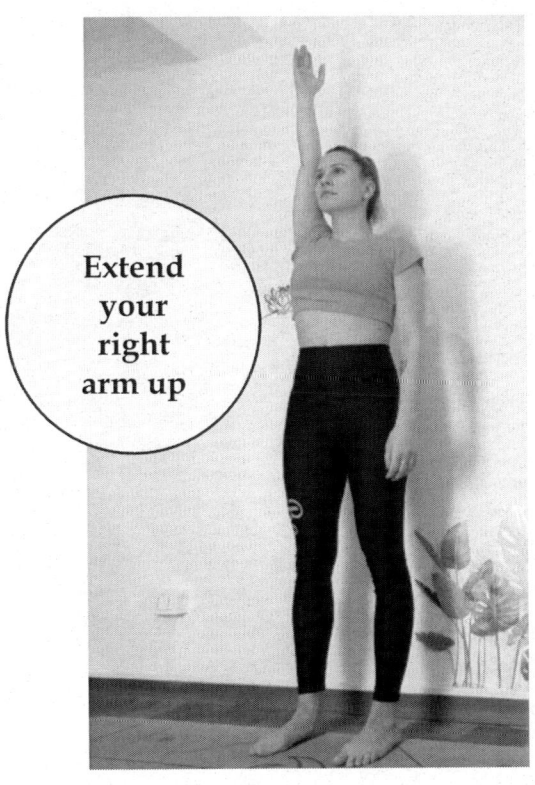

Extend your right arm up

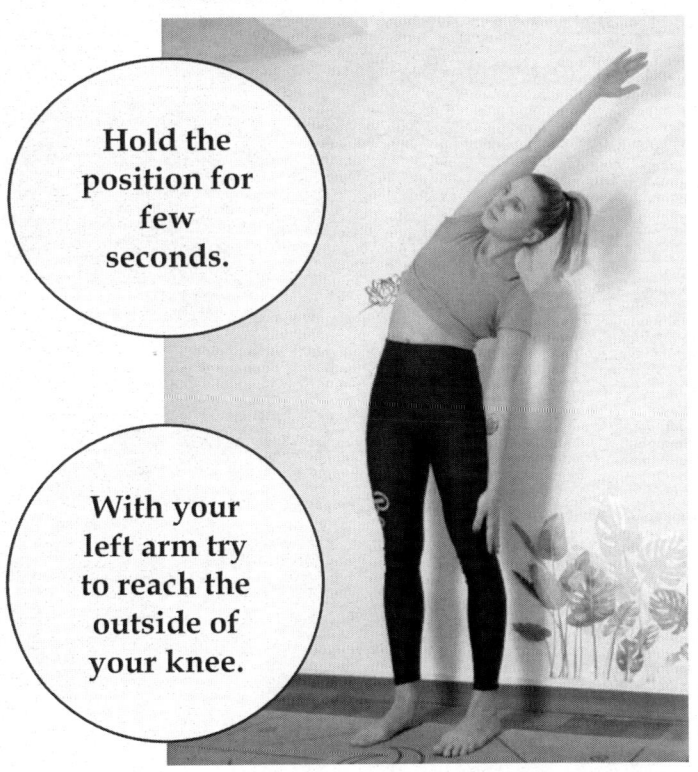

Hold the position for few seconds.

With your left arm try to reach the outside of your knee.

Pandiculation: Exercise 4 for Shoulder and Neck

Benefits

Last proposed exercise to release the accumulated stress and tension in the shoulders and neck.

Instructions

1. Stand with your back flat and feet hip - width apart.

2. bring the right shoulder forward and the left shoulder back.

3. Roll the palm in of the right arm.

4. Roll the palm of the left arm to face out behind you.

5. Twist the body and your head.

TIP: Let the head twist just enough to find a pleasurable stretch.

6. Hold the position for a couple of seconds, then slowly twist back your head and back in the starting position.

7. Repeat the stretch on the opposite side.

Breathing

Inhale before starting the stretch.

Exhale to twist.

Repetitions, Sets, and Rest

10 repetitions for 1 – 2 sets, resting for 30 seconds between each set.

Suitable for

Relieve stress and tension in the shoulders and neck.

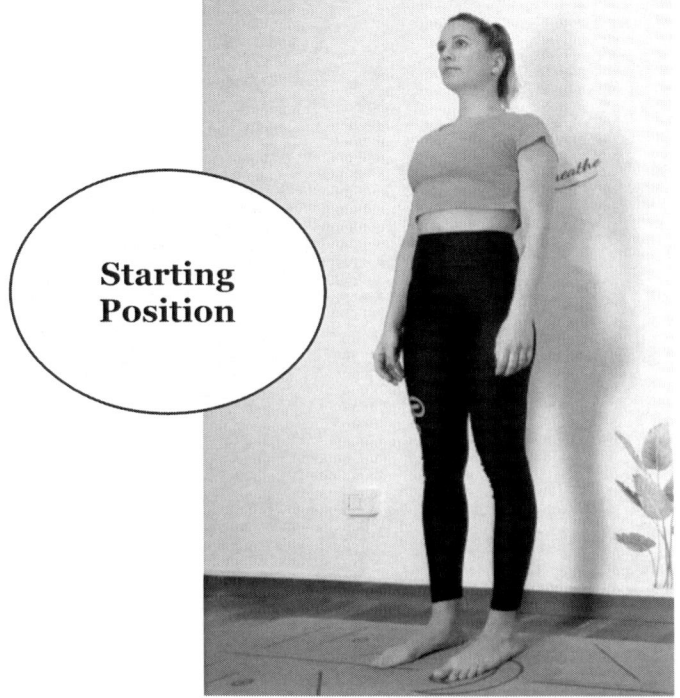

Starting Position

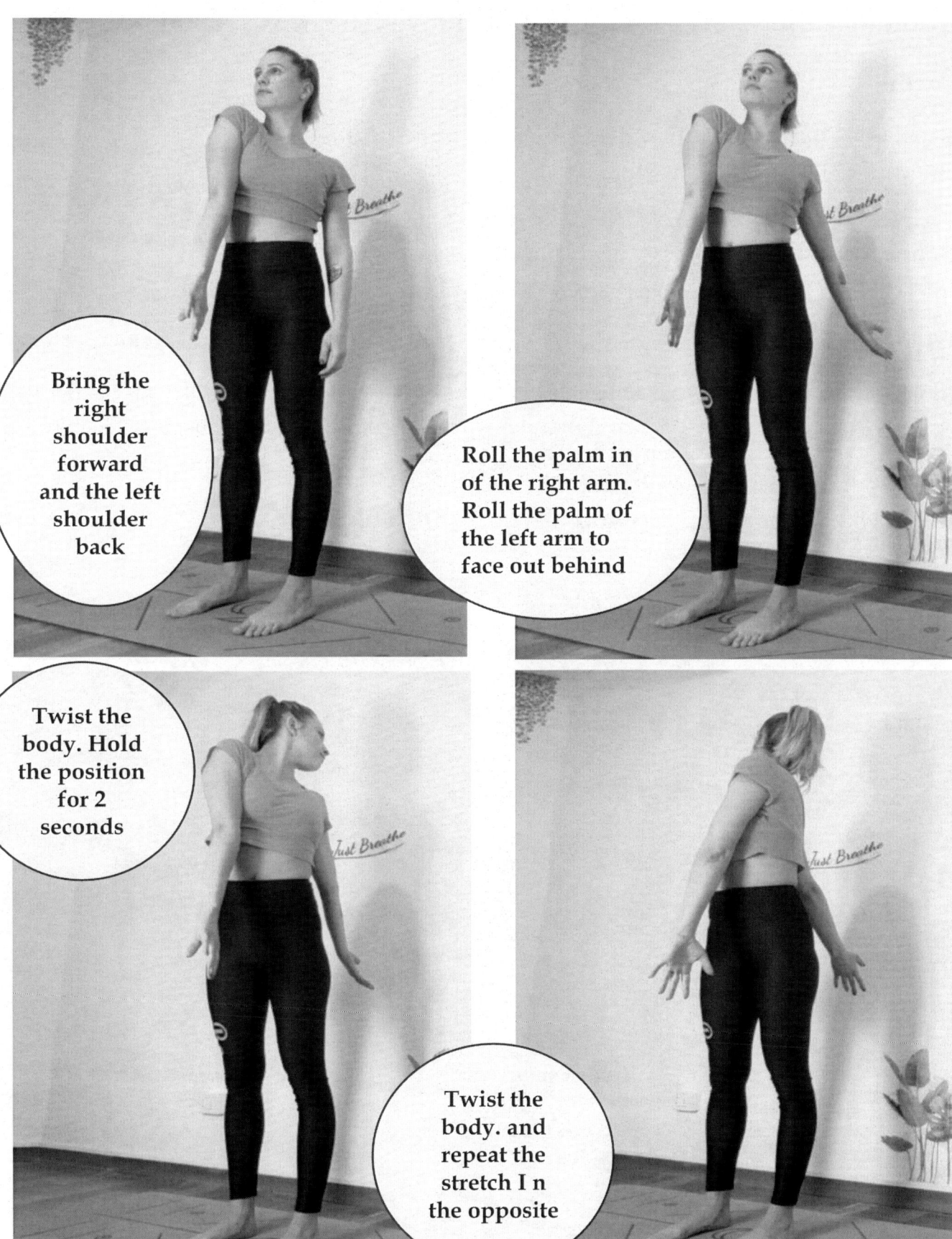

Pandiculation: Exercise 1 for Psoas - Flexes the hips

Benefits

The psoas is a major muscle that affects posture, flexibility, and joint function, particularly in the hips and lower back. This first proposed exercise focuses on improving Hip Flexibility, and alleviates hips pain.

Instructions

1. Stand straight with your back flat and feet hip width apart.

2. Take a small step forward with your right leg and lift up your left knee towards your chest.

3. Step back to the starting position and repeat with the other leg.

Breathing

Inhale while stepping forward.

Exhale to lift up the knee.

Repetitions, Sets, and Rest

20 repetitions alternating legs, for 3 sets, resting for 30 seconds between each set.

Suitable for

Improve hips flexibility.

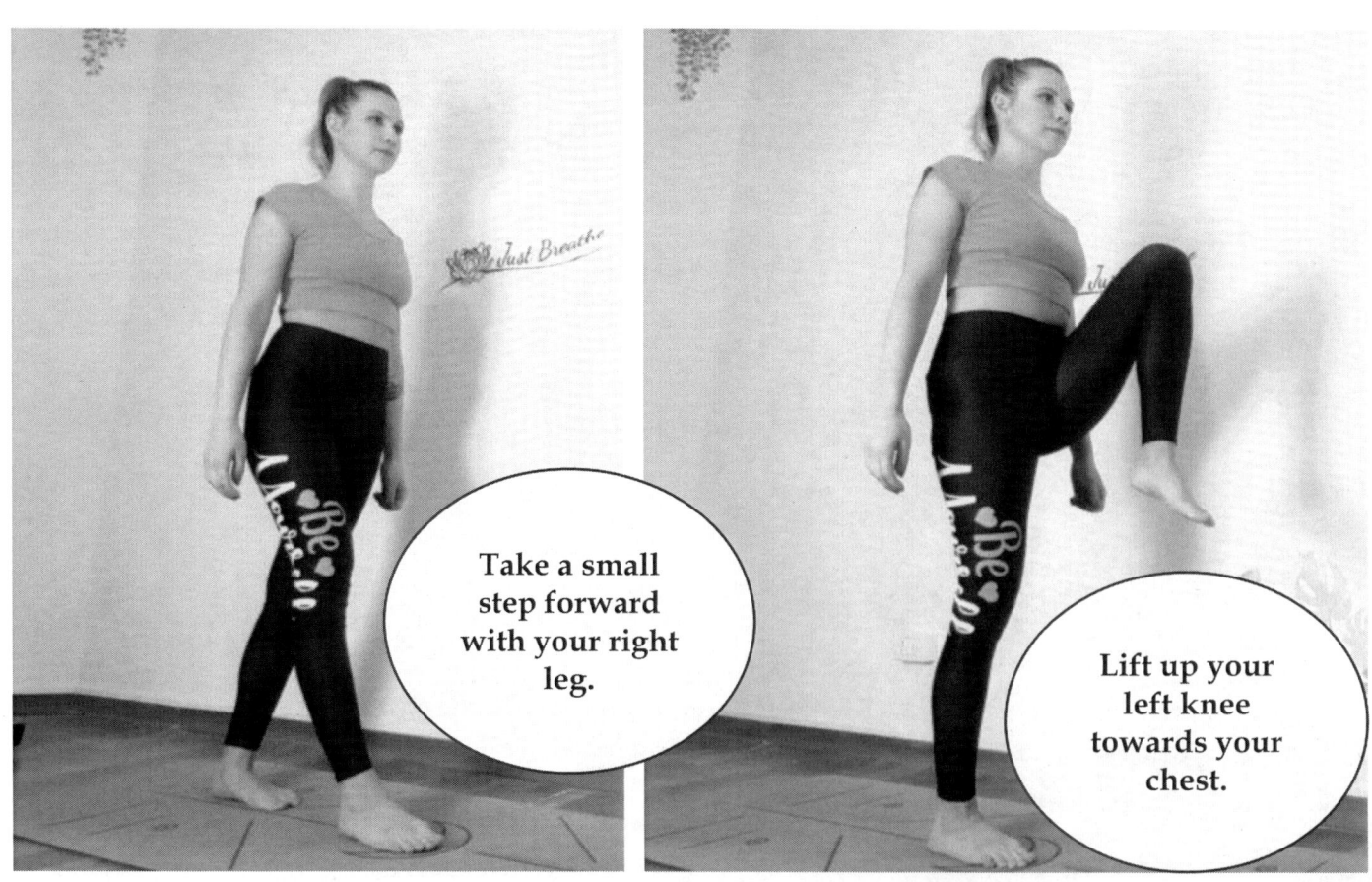

Take a small step forward with your right leg.

Lift up your left knee towards your chest.

Pandiculation: Exercise 2 for Psoas - Adducts the hips

Benefits

This second proposed exercise focuses on activating and engaging the hips muscles involved in the movement.

ips tension

Instructions

1. Lie down on your back. Keep your core tight and your back glued to the floor.

Tip: Pay attention to the back position: avoid to arch it.

2. Lift your legs up and perform a scissor movement with your legs.

Tip: To make it easier for your core muscles, lift your legs higher.

Breathing

Inhale and Exhale normally during the exercise.

Repetitions and Sets

2 – 3 sets. Rest 30 – 60 seconds each set.

Suitable for

Activate and engage the hips.

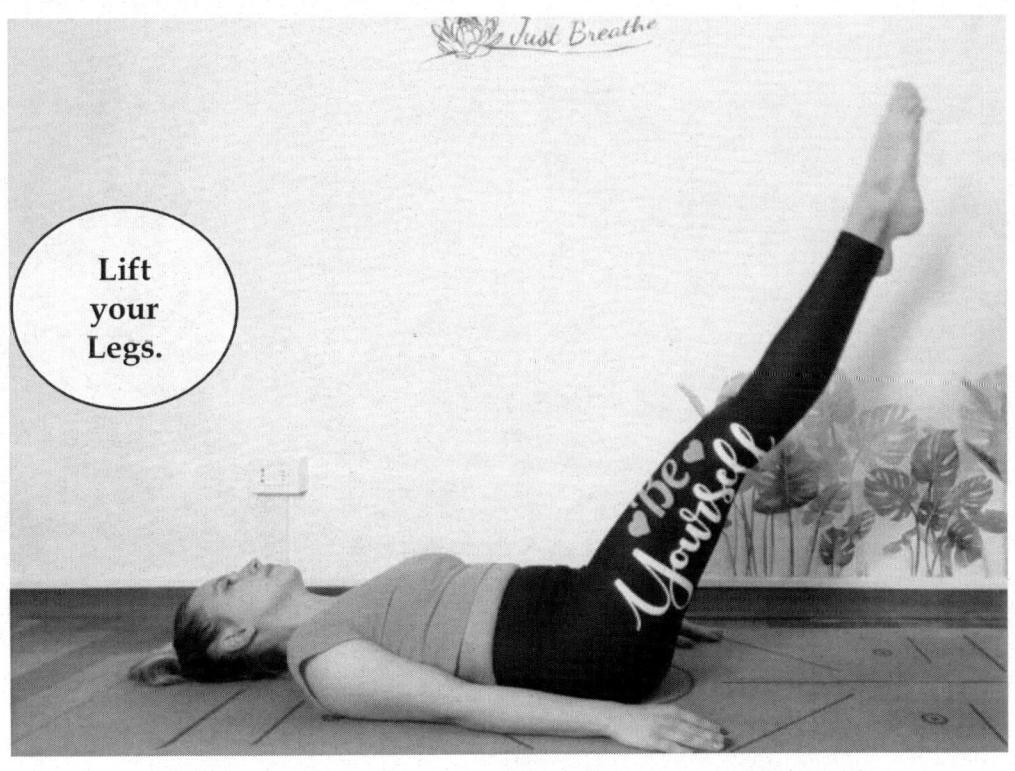

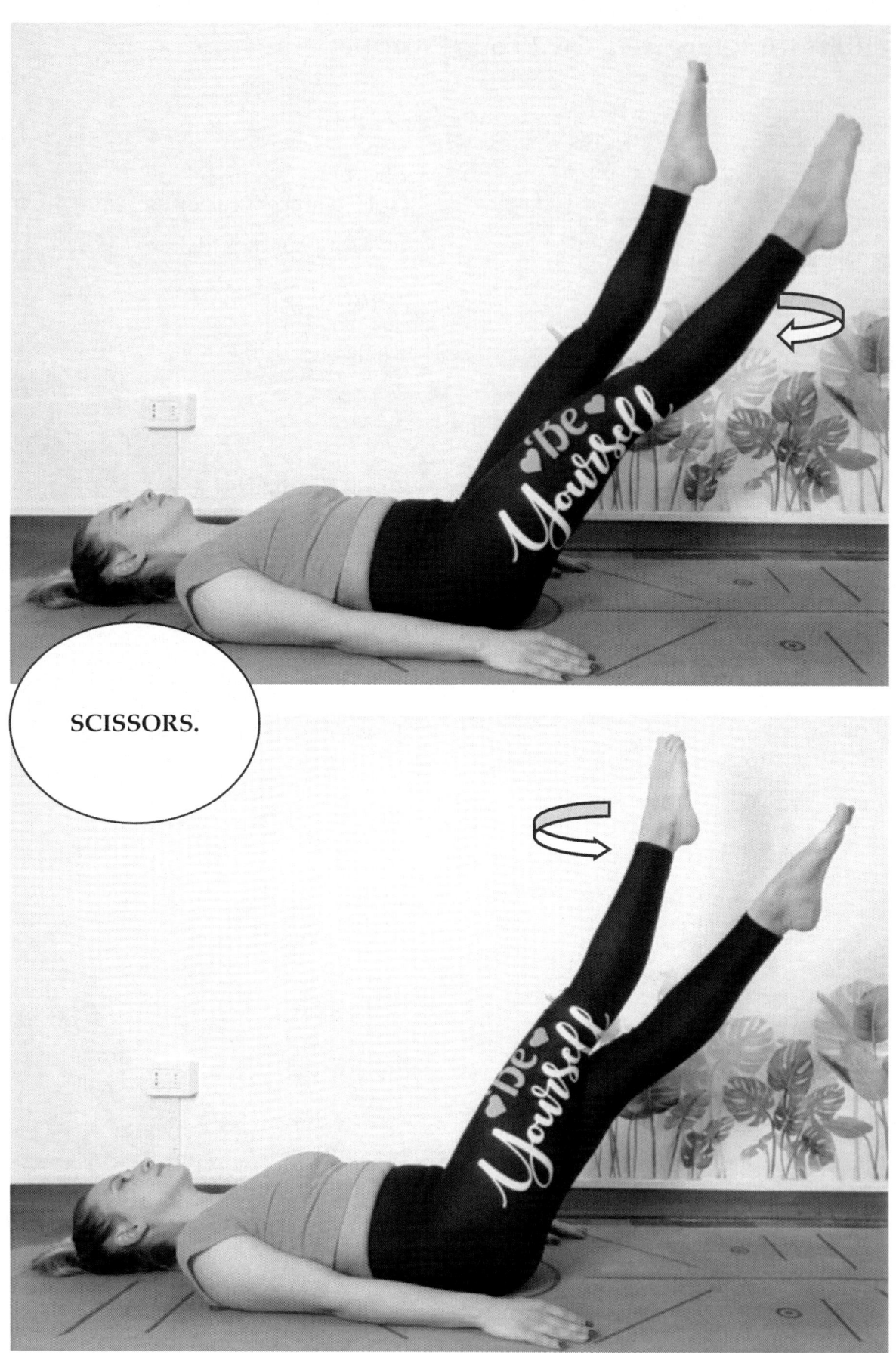

SCISSORS.

Pandiculation: Exercise 3 for Psoas - Laterally tilts the Pelvis

Benefits

This third proposed exercise strengthens the abductor muscles, enhances core stability, and functional movements.

Instructions

1. Stand with your back straight, chest open and shoulders down, arms by your sides. Now gently lift your right hip up.

2. Hold for a couple of seconds then release down.

3. Repeat with the other hip.

Breathing

Inhale in neutral position.

Exhale to lift the hip up.

Repetitions and Sets

10 repetitions alternating the hips for 1 – 2 sets, resting 30 seconds each set.

Suitable for

Enhance core stability.

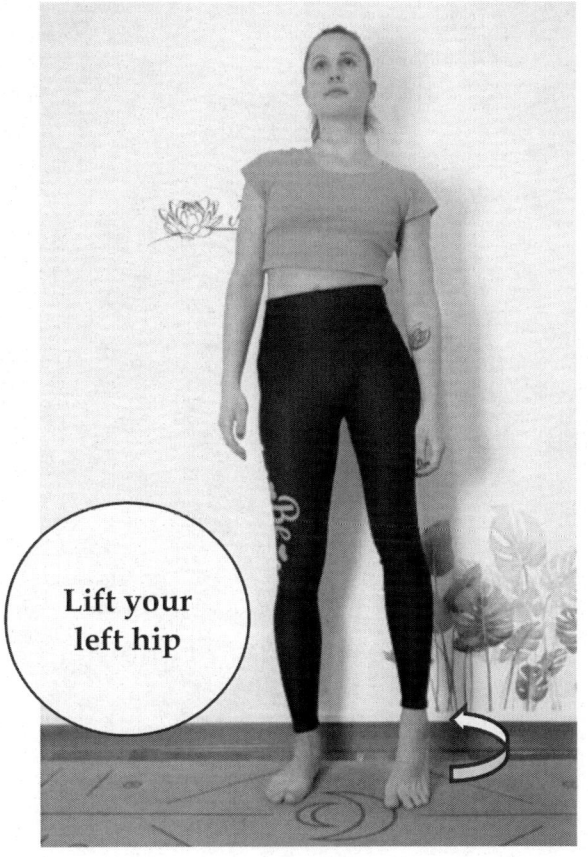

Lift your right hip

Lift your left hip

Pandiculation: Exercise 4 for Psoas - Laterally Flexes the Spine

Benefits

This fourth proposed exercise is excellent for balancing and strengthening the oblique muscles, and improving spinal mobility.

Instructions

1. Lift your right arm up.

2. Bend your upper body to the left, keeping your right arm fully extended and your left arm with the elbow at a 90-degree angle.

3. Keep the position for few seconds.

Breathing

Inhale and lift your right arm up.

Exhale and bend your upper body to the left.

Repetitions, Sets, and Rest

10 repetitions alternating sides for 1 – 2 sets, resting 30 seconds each set.

Suitable for

Obliques muscles balance and strengthen.

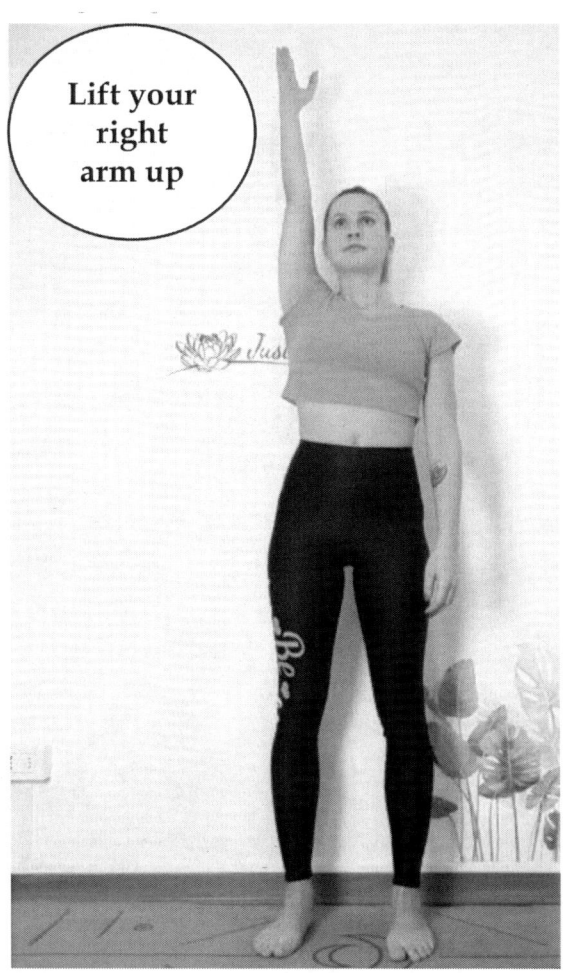

Lift your right arm up

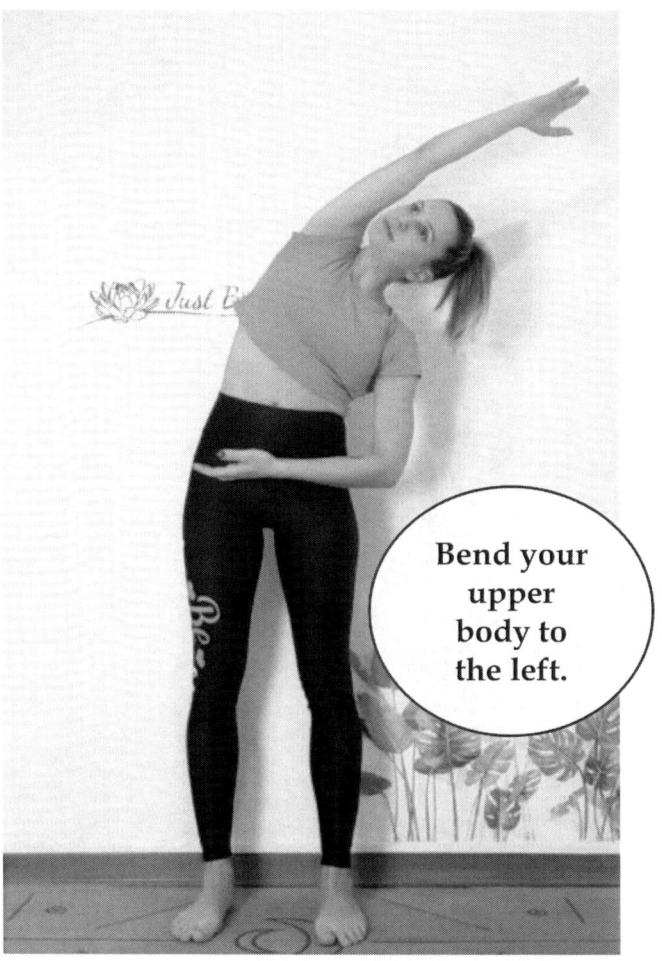

Bend your upper body to the left.

Pandiculation: Exercise 5 for Psoas - Release Arch and Flatten

Benefits

This last exercise is excellent to improving posture, reducing lower back pain, Enhancing Spinal Mobility, improving breathing mechanics, and enhancing body awareness.

Instructions – Arch Release

1. Line your back with your knees bent and your feet in line with your hips.

TIP: You can rest your arms by your sides on the floor or let your palms rest on your belly to bring awareness to your breath.

2. Gently roll your pelvis arching your lower back and sticking out your belly. Your tailbone will remain on the floor.

3. Back to the starting position without engaging your abdominal muscles.

4. Lift your right knee toward your chest, avoiding any tilting in your hips.

5. Lower your knee with a controlled a fluid movement.

6. Repeat the exercise using your left knee.

TIP: Adjust the difficulty by changing the distance between your feet and the wall.

Breathing

Inhale down into your belly and gently roll your pelvis.

Exhale and slowly release your lower back muscles.

Instructions – Flattening

1. Flatten your lower back down into the floor using your abdominal muscles.

TIP: Try to get the feeling of hollowing out your belly.

2. Release your abdominal muscles. slowly and back to the starting position.

Breathing

Inhale down into your belly allowing your abdominal muscles to relax and your lower belly to expand.

Exhale as you flatten your lower back down into the floor.

Repetitions, Sets, and Rest

10 repetitions (arch and flatten) for 2 – 3 sets, resting 30 seconds each set.

Suitable for

Posture improving.

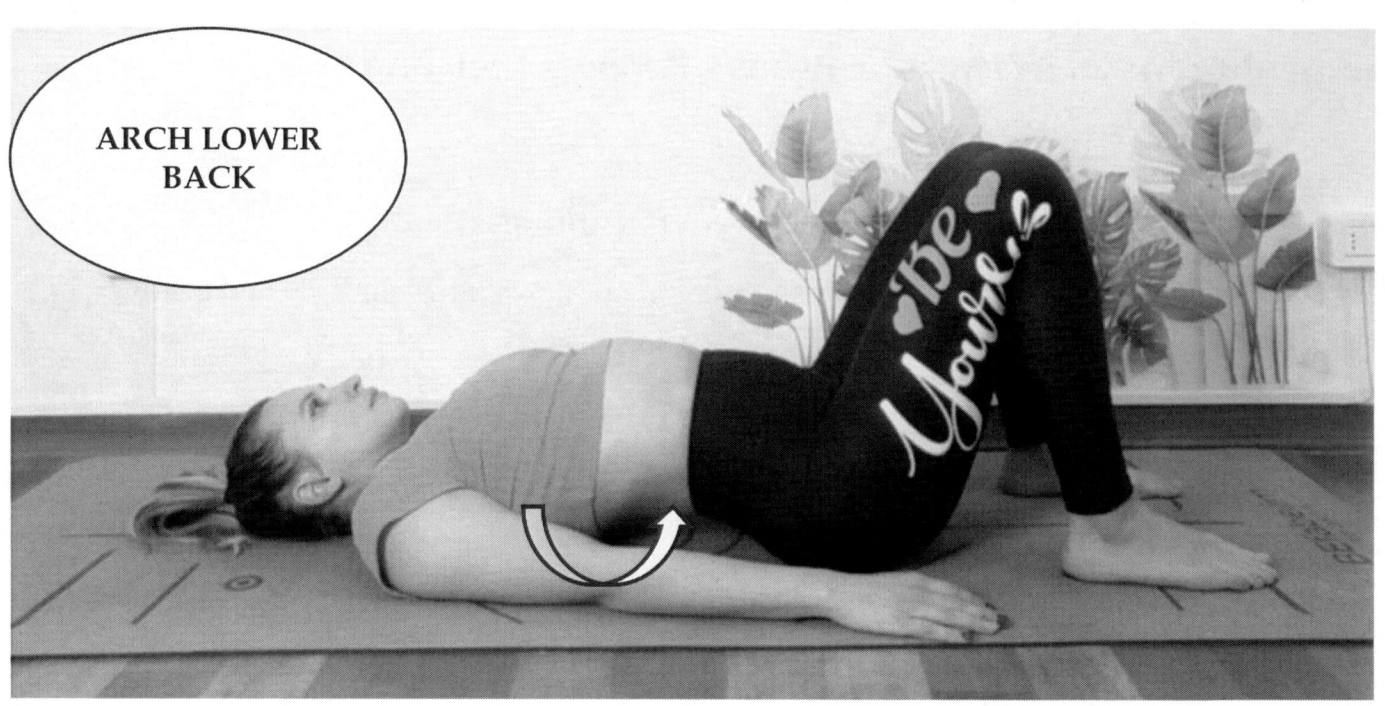

ARCH LOWER
BACK

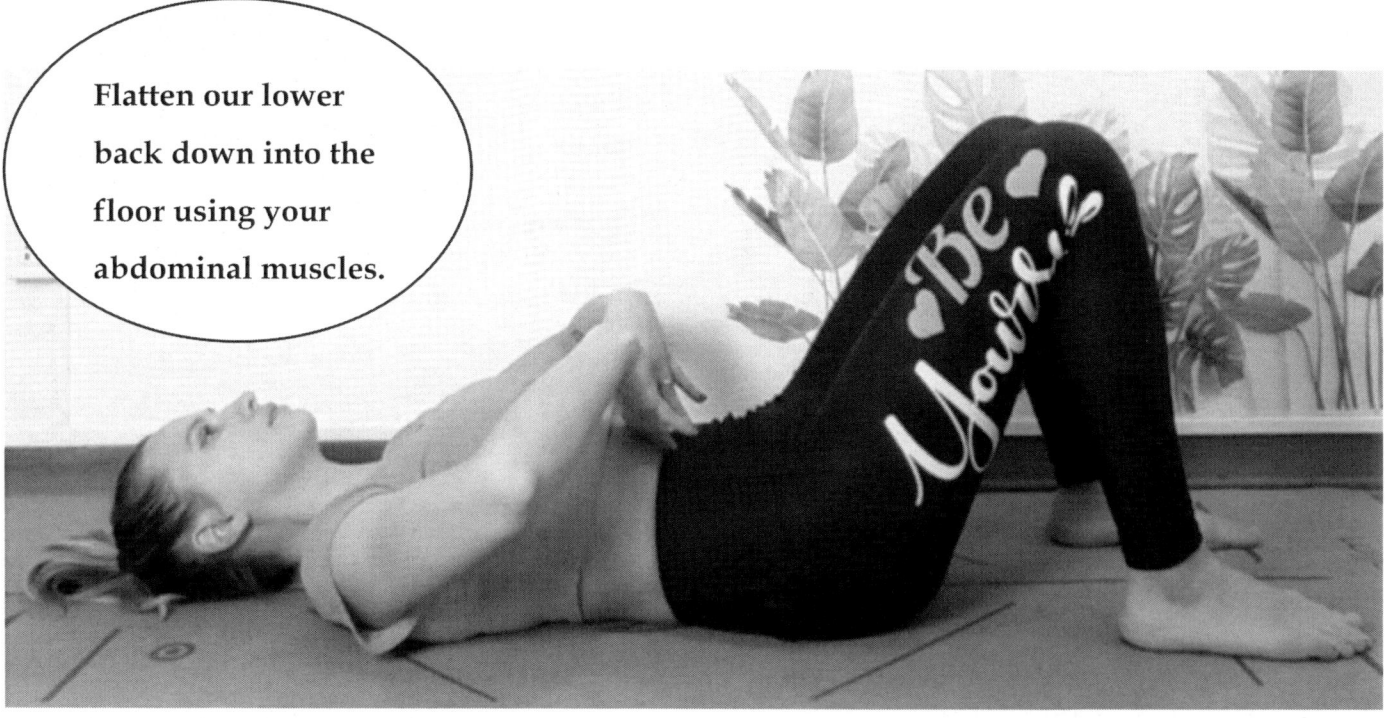

Flatten our lower
back down into the
floor using your
abdominal muscles.

Cat Cow Stretch

Benefits

This exercise promotes spinal mobility and postural awareness. It's excellent for enhancing digestion, alleviating back pain, improving circulation, and providing stress relief.

Instructions

1. Start in a tabletop position with your knees directly below your hips and your wrists and elbows are in line with your shoulders, your neck long, eyes looking at the floor.

2. Cow Pose: drop down your belly, lift your chin and chest and gaze up towards the ceiling .

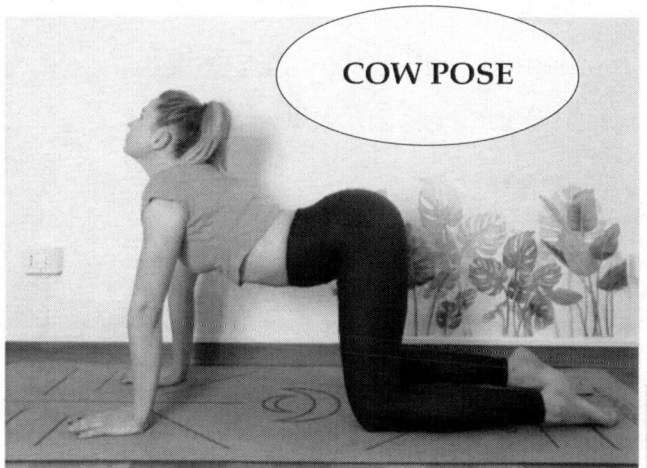

COW POSE

3. Cat Pose:.draw your belly to the spine and round your back towards the ceiling. Gently bring your chin to chest.

Breathing

Inhale into Cow Pose.

Exhale into Cat Pose.

Repetitions and Sets

Fluid *Cow and Cat* Movements for 1 -2 minutes.

Suitable for

Enhance the spinal mobility and postural awareness.

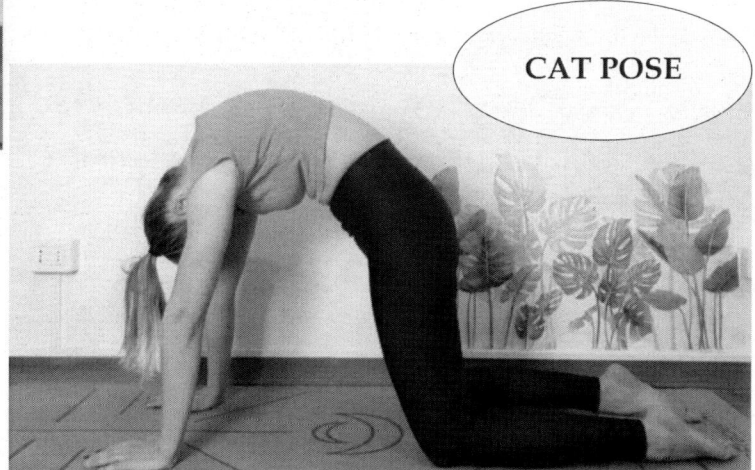

CAT POSE

Breathwork

Somatic breathwork is a practice that combines principles of somatic experiencing and conscious breathing techniques to promote relaxation, release tension, and enhance overall well-being. It involves using the breath as a tool to connect with and regulate the body's physiological responses, with the goal of fostering greater awareness, presence, and embodiment.

In somatic breathwork, you will explore your breath patterns and bodily sensations, paying close attention to the way breath moves through different parts of the body. By consciously directing the breath into areas of tension or discomfort, you can facilitate the release of physical and emotional holding patterns, promoting a sense of ease and relaxation.

Somatic breathwork incorporates various breathing techniques, such as deep diaphragmatic breathing, rhythmic breathing, or breathwork exercises derived from pranayama (yogic breathing practices). These techniques are used to regulate the nervous system, balance energy, and induce states of relaxation or arousal as needed.

Main Benefits of somatic breathwork

Stress Reduction: Conscious breathing techniques activates the body's relaxation response, reducing levels of stress hormones and promoting a sense of calm and well-being.

Emotional Regulation: By bringing awareness to the breath and bodily sensations, it develops greater emotional resilience and regulation skills, helping you manage difficult emotions more effectively.

Increased Body Awareness: Somatic breathwork encourages routinely practitioners to tune into their bodies and cultivate greater awareness of physical sensations, promoting a deeper connection to the present moment and fostering a sense of embodiment.

Improved Mental Clarity: Breathwork practices can help clear the mind, increase focus, and enhance mental clarity, providing a valuable tool for managing overwhelm or racing thoughts.

Overall, somatic breathwork offers a holistic approach to well-being, addressing the interconnectedness of mind, body, and breath

Breathwork: Exercise 1 - Seated Pose

Benefits

This exercise is very useful to feel your grounded and centered. It facilitates breath awareness and emotional regulation.

Instructions

1. Sit comfortably on a chair. Bring your left hand behind your head and leave the right arm hanging down.

2. Length your spine and gently bend your head to the right.

3. Stretch your right arm, then bring back your head to the starting position.

4. Repeat the exercise with the other hand.

Breathing

Inhale before bending your head and as you stretch your arms over your head.

Exhale as you bend your head and as you bring it back to the starting position.

Repetitions and Sets

10 –repetitions each arm.

Suitable for

Facilitate emotional regulation and breath awareness.

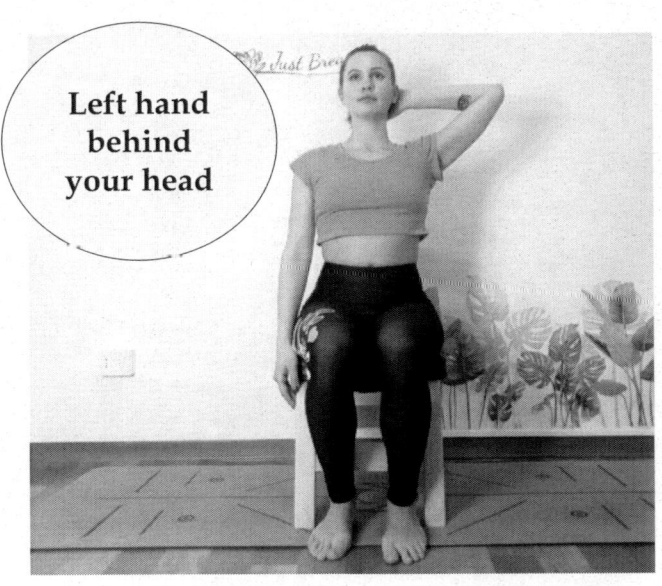

Left hand behind your head

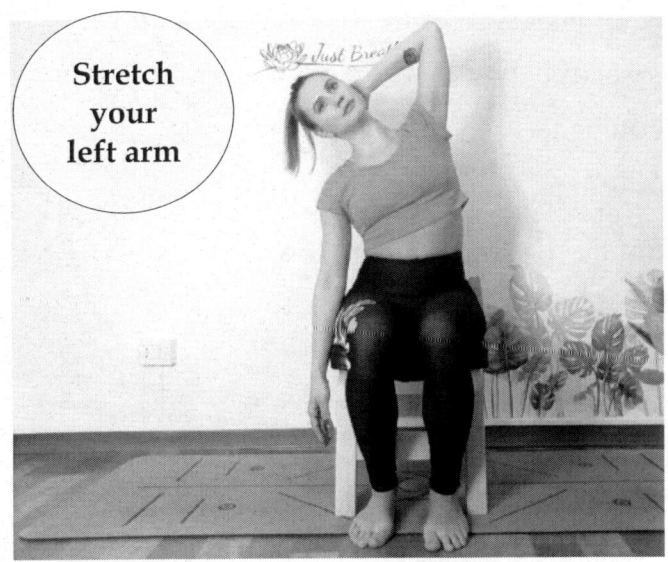

Stretch your left arm

Breathwork: Exercise 2 – Diaphragmatic Breathing

Benefits

This exercise focuses on engaging the diaphragm muscle to facilitate deep, belly breathing while maintaining an upright posture. It helps improve posture, promote relaxation, and enhance breath awareness while standing.

Instructions

1. Stand upright with feet shoulder -width apart and knees slightly bent for stability. Place one hand on the middle of your upper chest and the other hand on the stomach, just beneath the rib cage.

Breathing

To Inhale: slowly breathe in through the nose, drawing the breath down towards the stomach.

To Exhale: tighten the abdominal muscles and let the stomach fall downward while exhaling through first lips.

TIP:

The stomach should push upward against the hand, while the chest remains still.

Repetitions and Sets

Practice this breathing exercise for 5 – 10 minutes at a time, for 3 – 4 times a day.

Suitable for

Engaging diaphragm muscle; improve posture; facilitate relaxation.

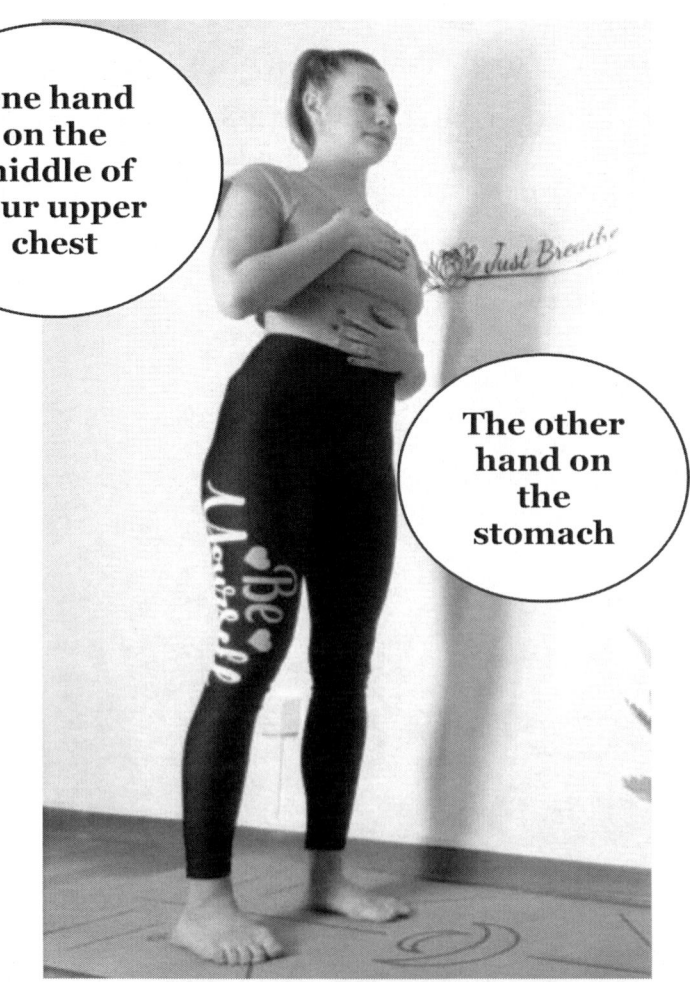

One hand on the middle of your upper chest

The other hand on the stomach

Breathwork: Exercise 3 – Diaphragmatic Breathing Supine

Benefits

In this exercise, you can use a flat surface such as a yoga mat or bed to facilitate the breathwork. It promotes relaxation, reduces muscle tension, and enhances breath awareness while lying in a reclined position.

Instructions

1. Lie down on your back. Legs extended. Under your knees place a rolled yoga mat, pillow, cushion or even fold a towel to make yourself comfortable and to facilitate the breathing practice.

2. Place one hand on the middle of your upper chest and the other hand on the stomach, just beneath the rib cage.

Breathing

To inhale: slowly breathe in through the nose drawing the breath down towards the stomach.

To exhale: tighten the abdominal muscles and let the stomach fold downward while exhaling through pursed lips.

TIP

The stomach should push upward against the hand, while the chest remains still.

Repetitions, Sets, and Rest

Practice this breathing exercise for 5 – 10 minutes at a time, for 3 – 4 times a day.

Suitable for

Engaging diaphragm muscle; improve posture; facilitate relaxation; enhance breath awareness.

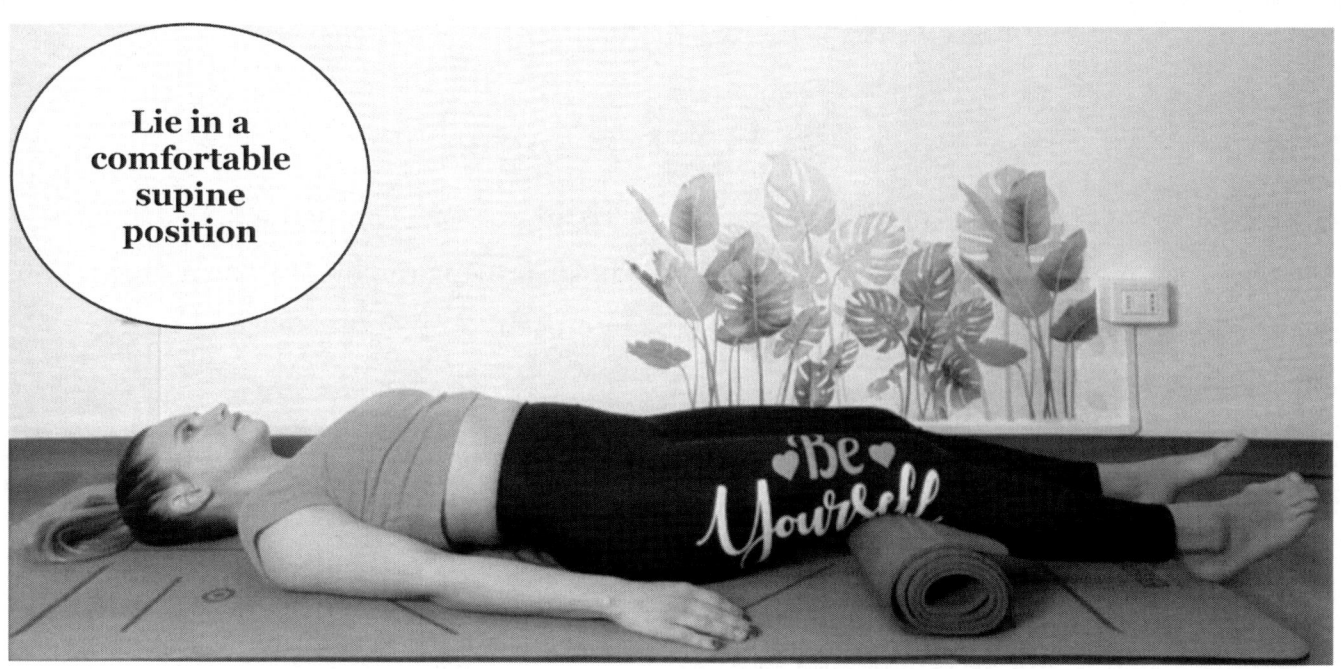

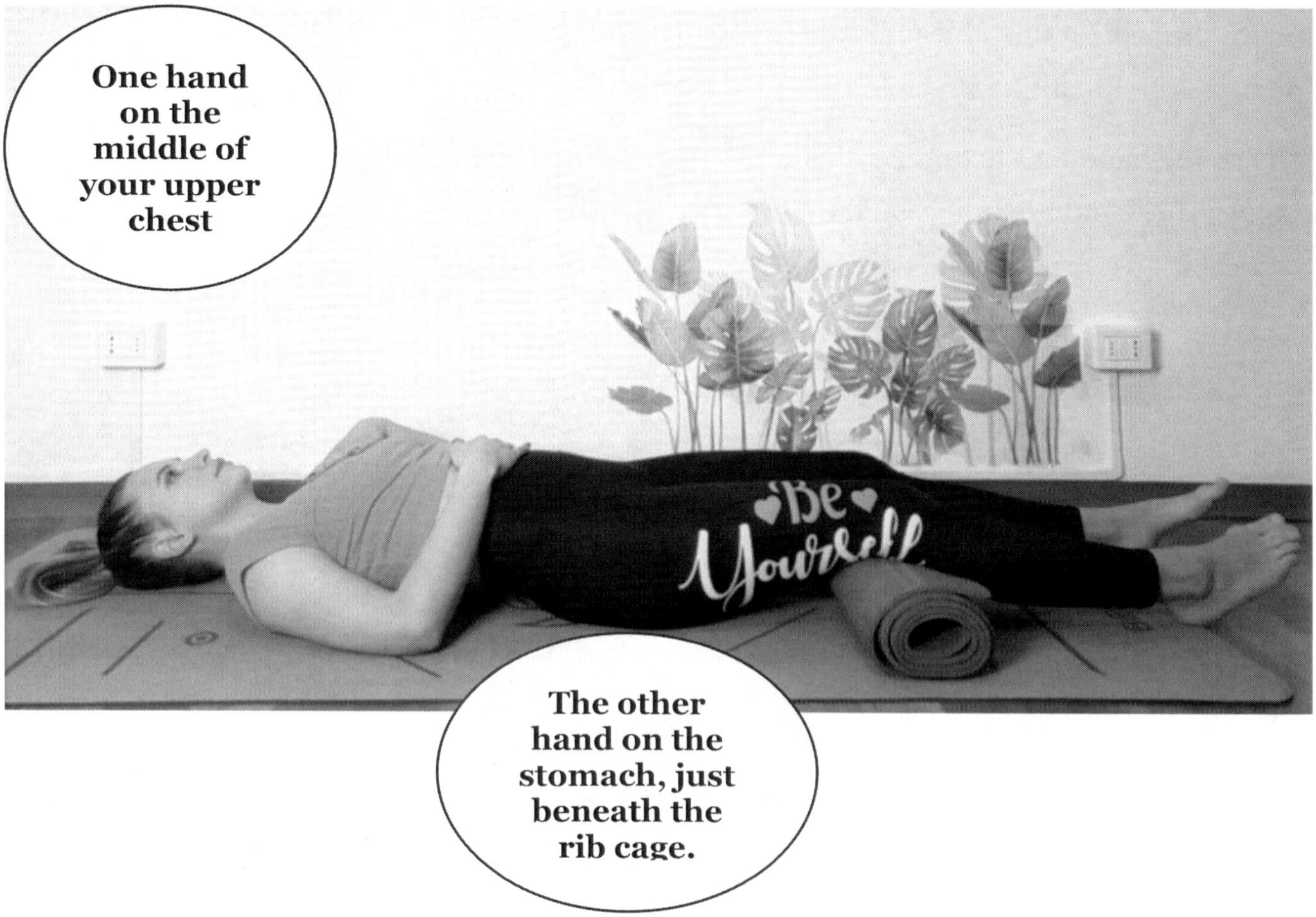

Breathwork: Exercise 4 – Breathing Techniques for Emotional Regulation

Benefits

This exercise increases emotional awareness and self-regulation. It facilitates the release of emotional and physical tension, as well as trauma, promoting emotional healing and integration.

Instructions

1. Sit comfortably with your legs crossed. Rest your hands on your knees, palms facing up or down, whichever you prefer.

Tip

Close your eyes if it feels good

Breathing

Inhale: count slowly from 1 to 4, matching your full inhale with the count 1, 2, 3, 4.

Hold your breath for a count 1 – 2.

Exhale: count slowly from 1 to 4 until your lungs are completely empty

Repetitions, Sets, and Rest

Practice the Breathing exercise for 5 – 10 minutes a day, and anytime you need to relax and regulate your emotional state.

Suitable for

Relax and regulate your emotional state.

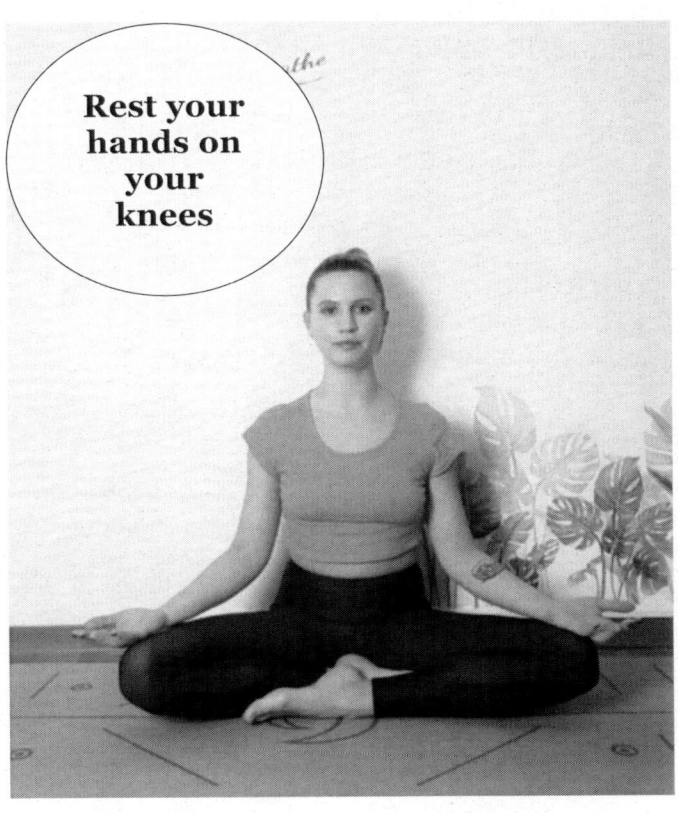

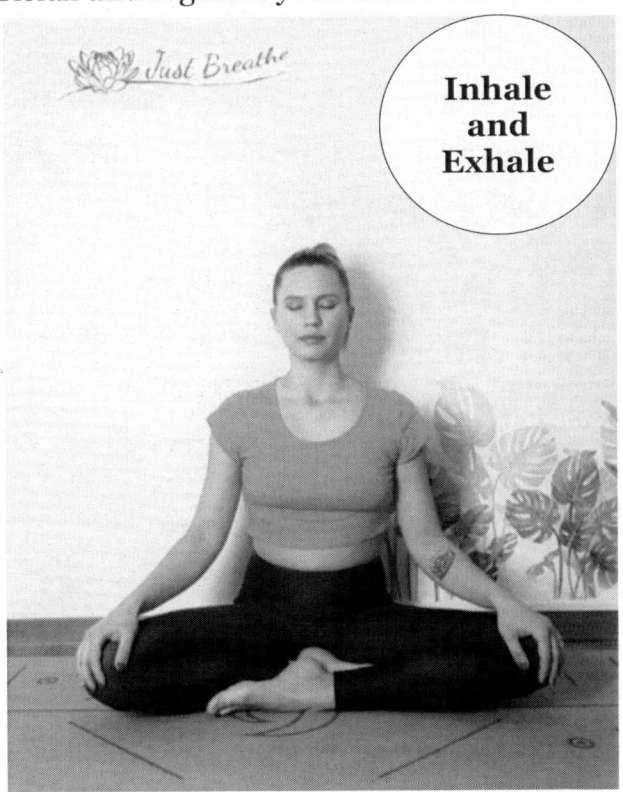

Breathwork: Exercise 5 – Breathing Techniques for Flexibility

Benefits

This exercise is very useful to prevent injury, joint mobility, and reduce the stress by inducing a deep state of relaxation in the body.

Instructions

1. Starting position: Sit down on your mat with your legs extended forward and your back straight.

2. Inhale and lift your arms up, then Exhale and bend your hips with your arms reaching forward into a folded position.

TIP

Keep your back as straight as possible.

3. Inhale and lift your arms up. Exhale and twist your body to the right, placing your fingertips on the floor.

4. Inhale and back to the starting position Exhale and twist your body to the left, placing your fingertips on the floor.

5. Lie down on your back, exhale as you bring your right knee to chest, hands clasped on the knee. Inhale and extend your right leg to the floor.

6. Exhale, and bring your left knee to chest, hands clasped on the knee.

Breathing

Inhale as you lift your arms up amd extend your legs.

Exhale as you bend your hips, twist your body, and bring your knee to the chest.

Repetitions, Sets, and Rest

Repeat the full breathing flexibility sequence 5 times for 2 – 5 sets, resting for 30 seconds each set.

Suitable for

Inducing a deep state of relaxation.

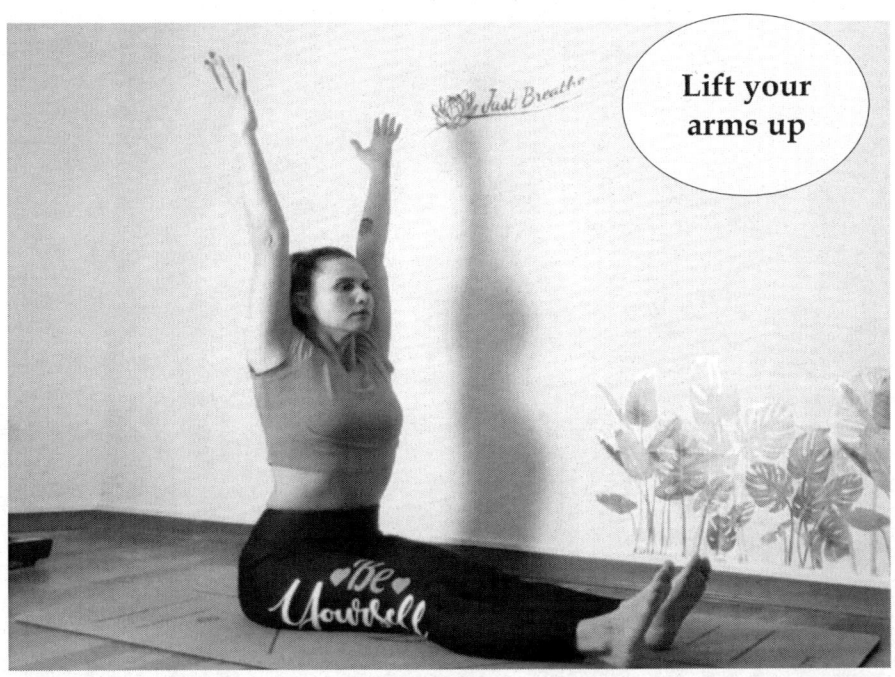

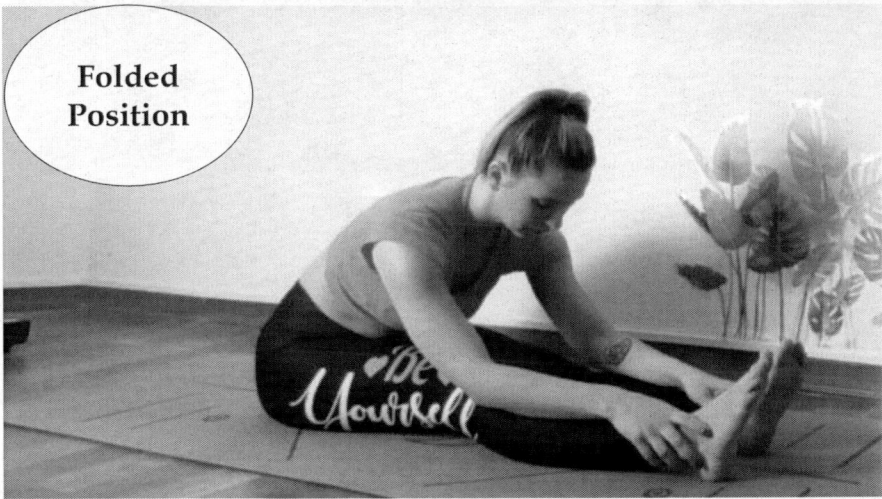

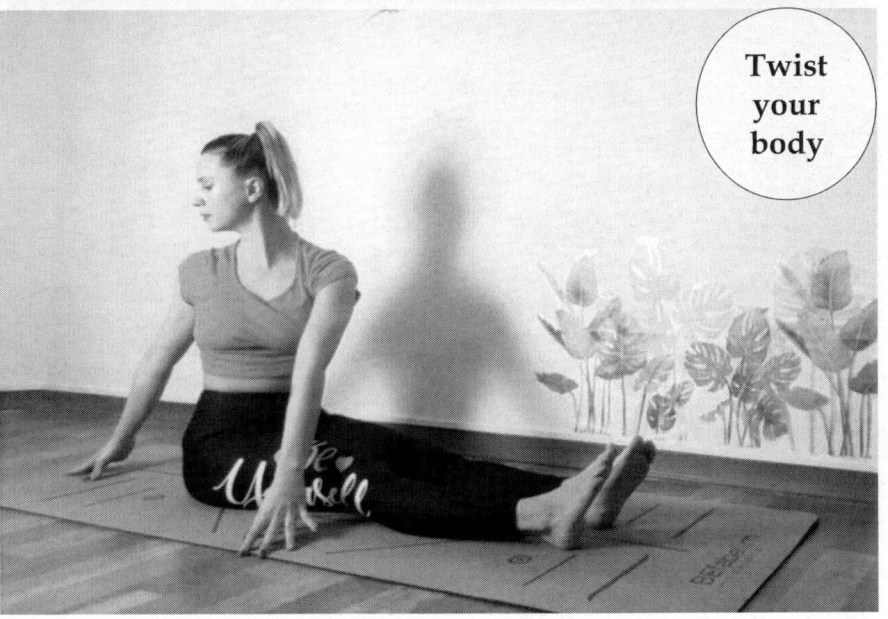

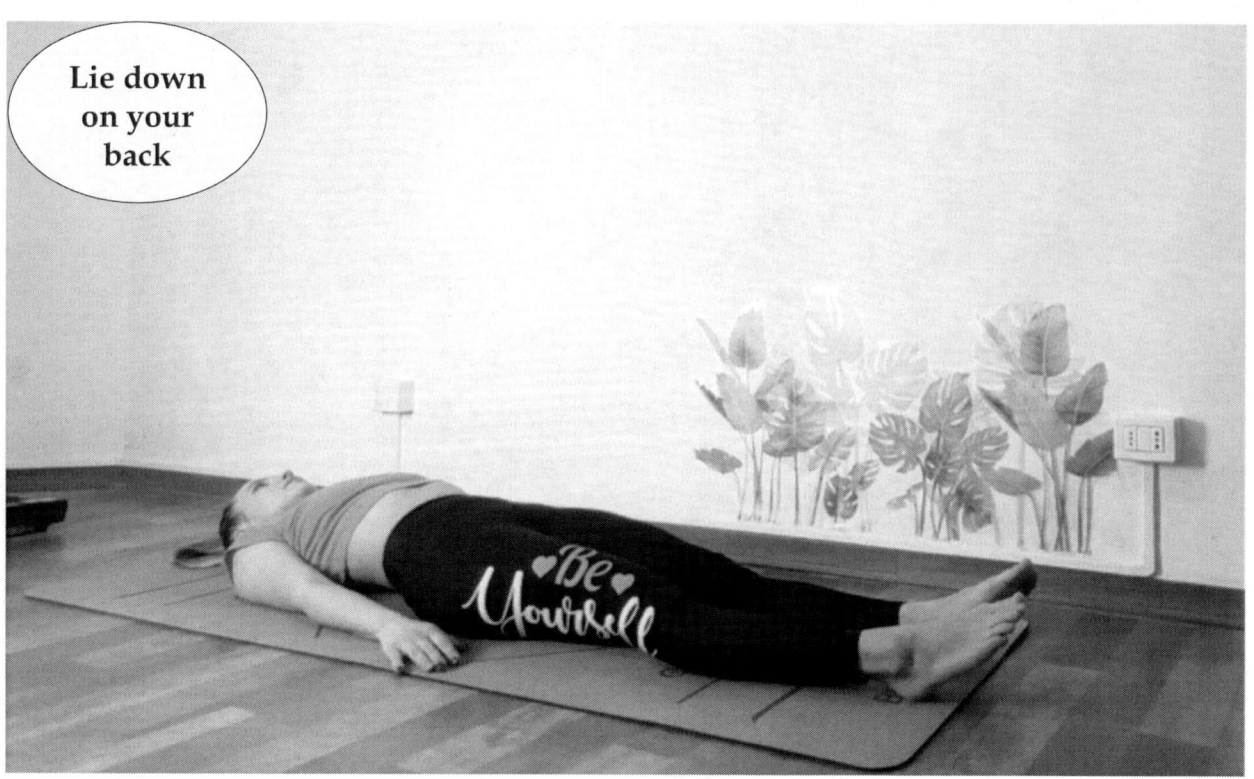

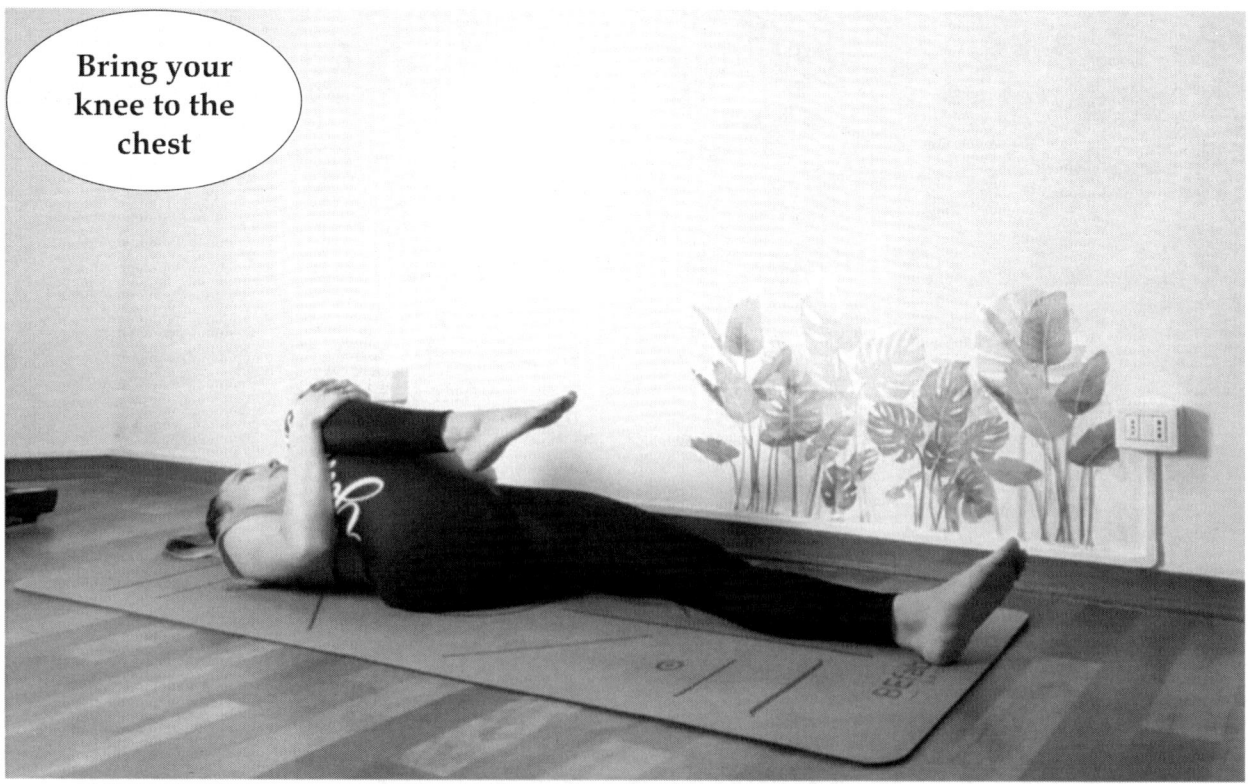

Breathwork: Exercise 6 – Alternate nostril Breathing

Benefits

This exercise improves oxygenation to muscles and tissues, and strongly enhances the mind/body connection by leading to greater awareness of sensations, including areas of tension or tightness.

Instructions

1. Sit in a comfortable position and rest your hands on your legs, palms facing up. Take your right hand. Make sure your index and middle finger are touching and bend them in towards the palm.

2. Take your right thumb and close your right nostril. Inhale through the left nostril, then place your ring and little finger against the left nostril as well.

3. Release the thumb and exhale through the right nostril. Inhale through the right and switch over and exhale through the left nostril.

4. Inhale through the left, swap the finger over, release the thumb and exhale out through the right. Then inhale through the right,

5. swap over, release the thumb and release the thumb. exhale through the left.

6. Breathe steady and calmly. Inhale and exhale throughout both nostrils to complete this breathing exercise.

Repetitions, Sets, and Rest

Repeat the exercise 10 – 20 times for 1 – 3 sets, resting for 45 – 60 seconds between each set.

Suitable for

Enhancing mind/ body connection and release tension or tightness.

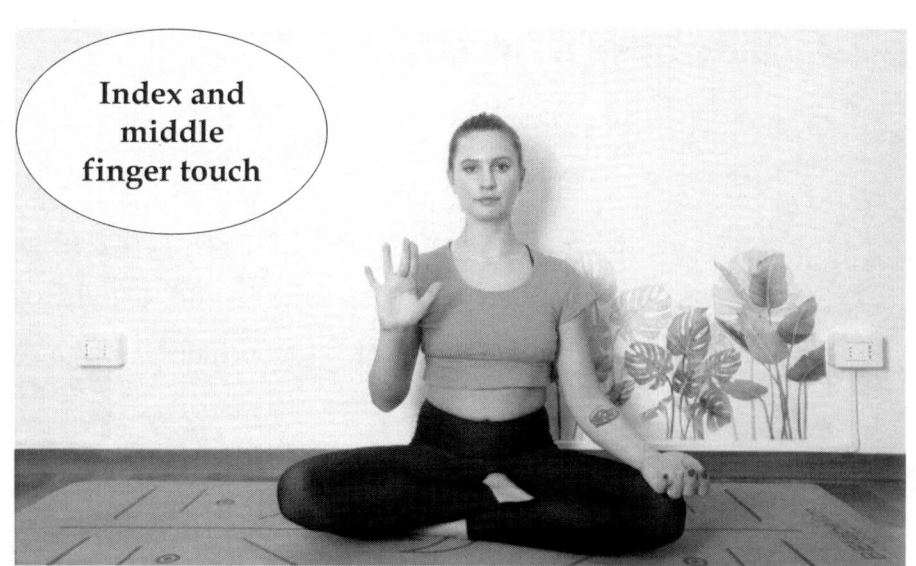

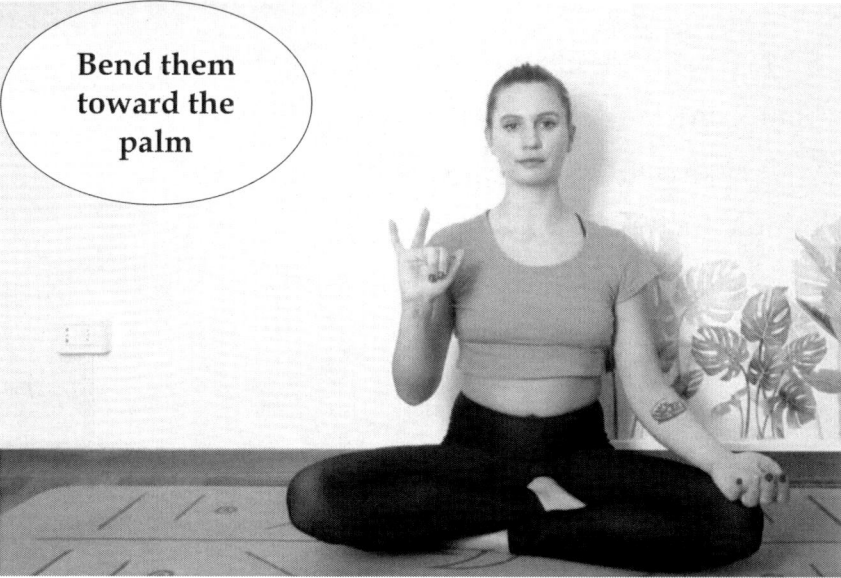

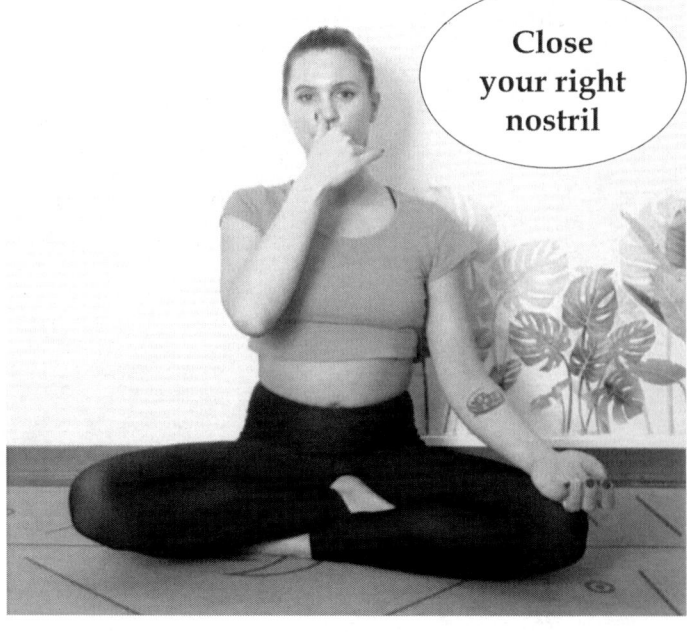

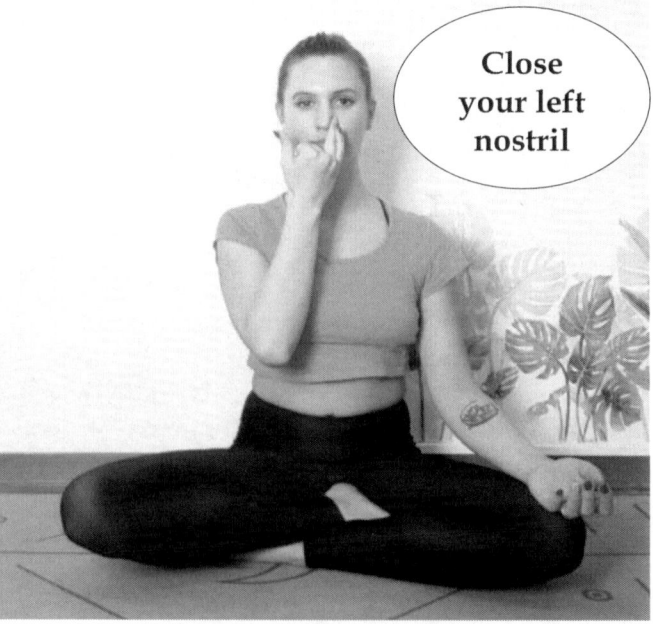

Movement Flow

Movement Flow: Exercise 1 – Release Tension and Trauma from the Hips

Benefits

This exercise releases accumulated tension in the muscles and tissues surrounding the hips. It is very useful for recovering from hip injuries or surgeries, as it gently mobilizes and strengthens the muscles in this area.

Instructions

1. Lie down on your back, arms by your sides. Bring the soles of your feet together and let your knees fall down to the sides into a reclined butterfly position.

2. Keep pressing your feet together and very slowly bring the knees towards each other.

Your legs might start shaking and releasing trauma and tension from the hips.

Breathing

Inhale as you are in the butterfly position.

Exhale to bring your knees together.

Repetitions, Sets, and Rest

5 repetitions for 2 – 3 sets, resting for 30 seconds each set.

Suitable for

Release tension and trauma from the hips.

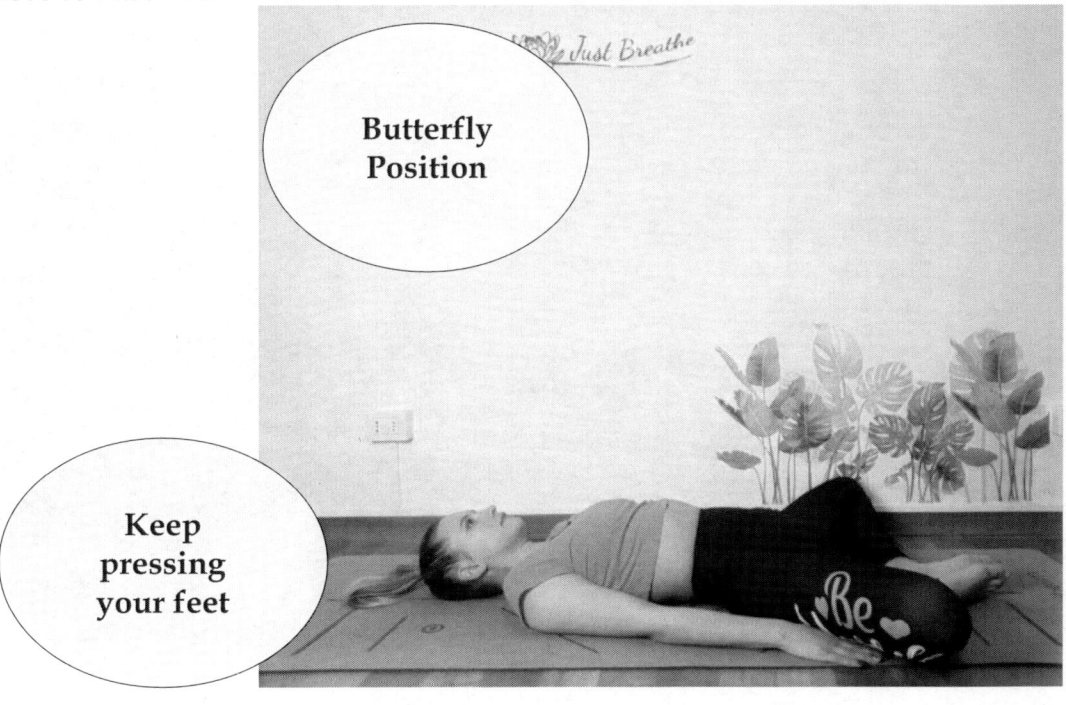

Butterfly Position

Keep pressing your feet

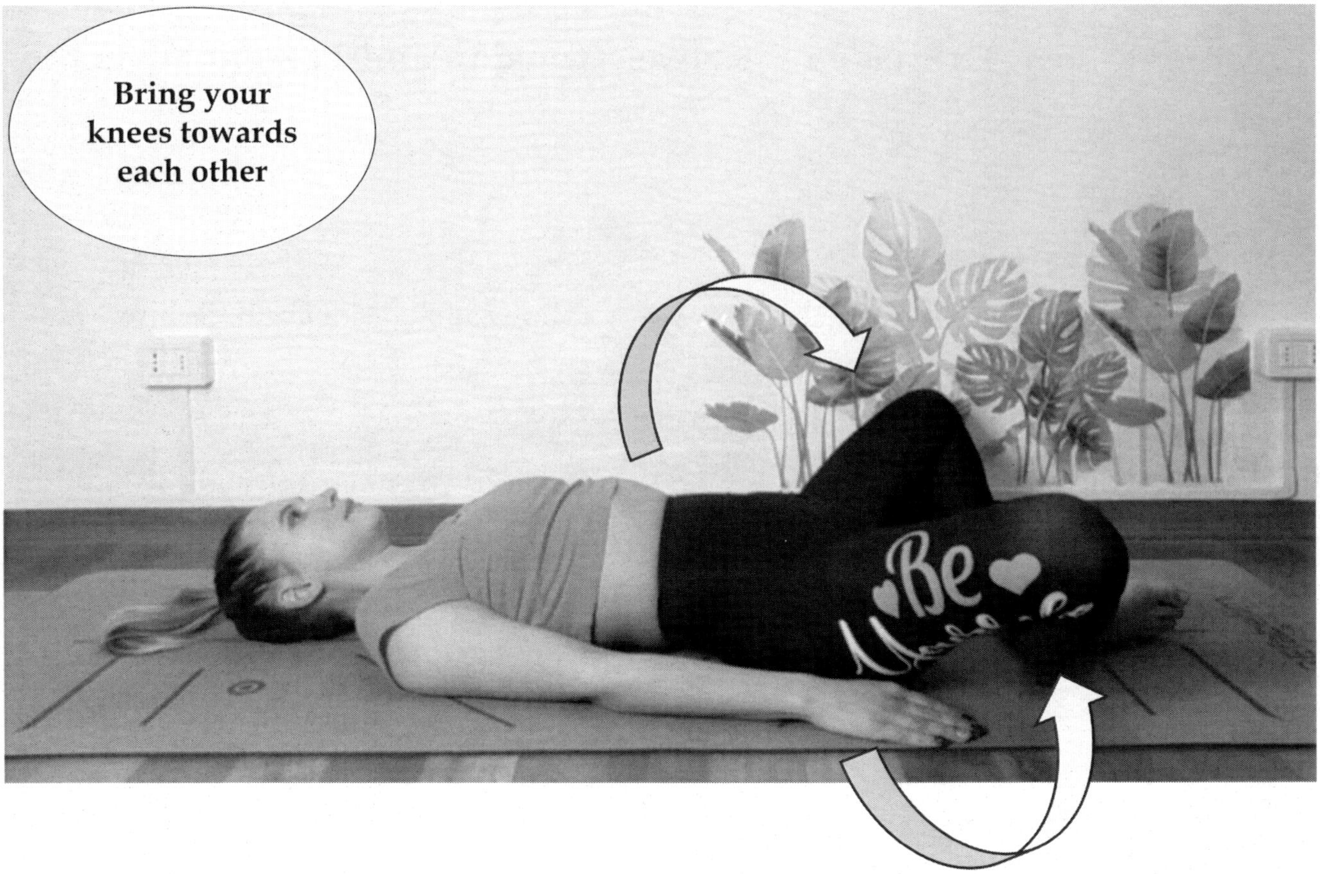

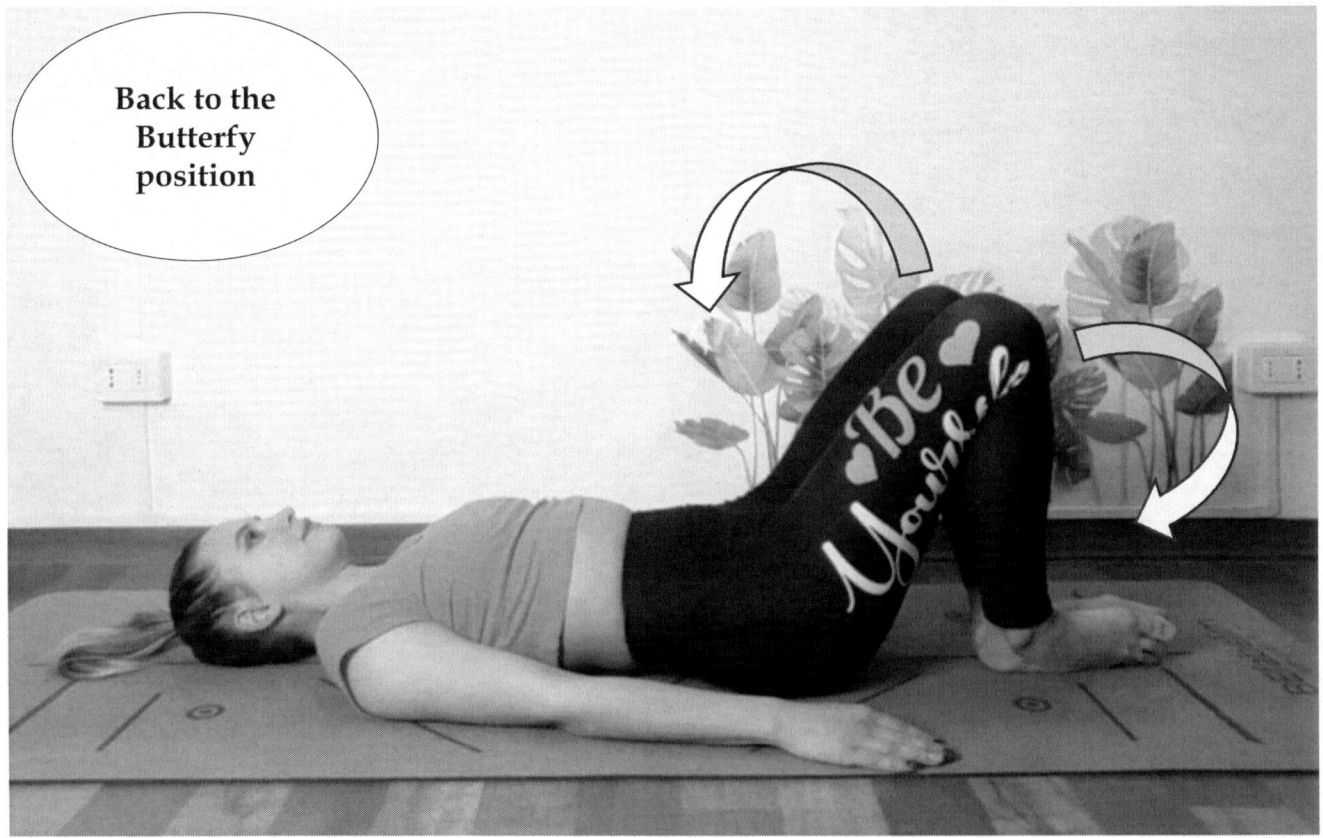

Movement Flow: Exercise 2 – Wrist Stretch

Benefits

Healthy wrists are essential for performing everyday tasks and activities with ease and comfort. This exercise enhances overall wrist health and function, supporting you in maintaining an active and fulfilling lifestyle.

Instructions

1. Sit onto your heels and open up your knees to the sides. Place your palms on the floor between your knees, fingers pointing backwards. Hold the position for about 60 seconds.

2. Turn your hands and put the backs of your hands on the ground. Hold the position for 60 seconds.

TIPS

While holding the positions 1. and 2., let your hands to peel up and come down.

You can gently shift your weight from side to side, lifting one hand at a time.

3. Release your arms: open and close the fingers repeatedly. Then circle your hands few times.

Breathing

Inhale and Exhale slowly during the exercise.

Repetitions, Sets, and Rest

Hold positions 1. and 2. for 60 seconds each.

Suitable for

Enhance overall wrist health and function.

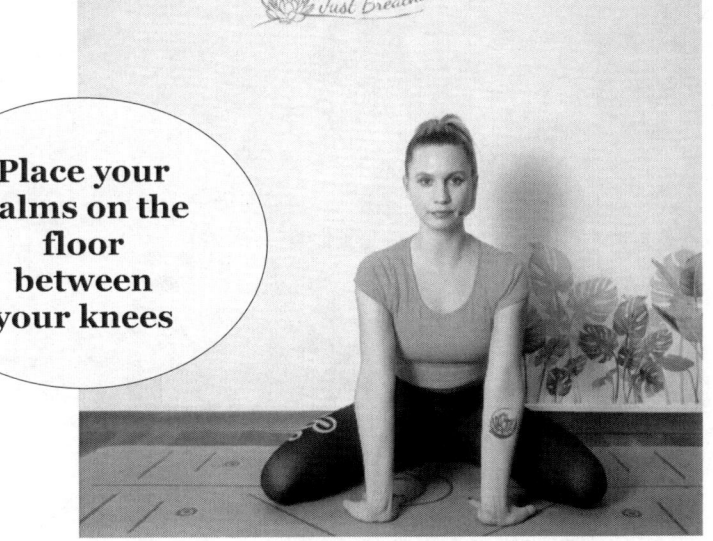

Place your palms on the floor between your knees

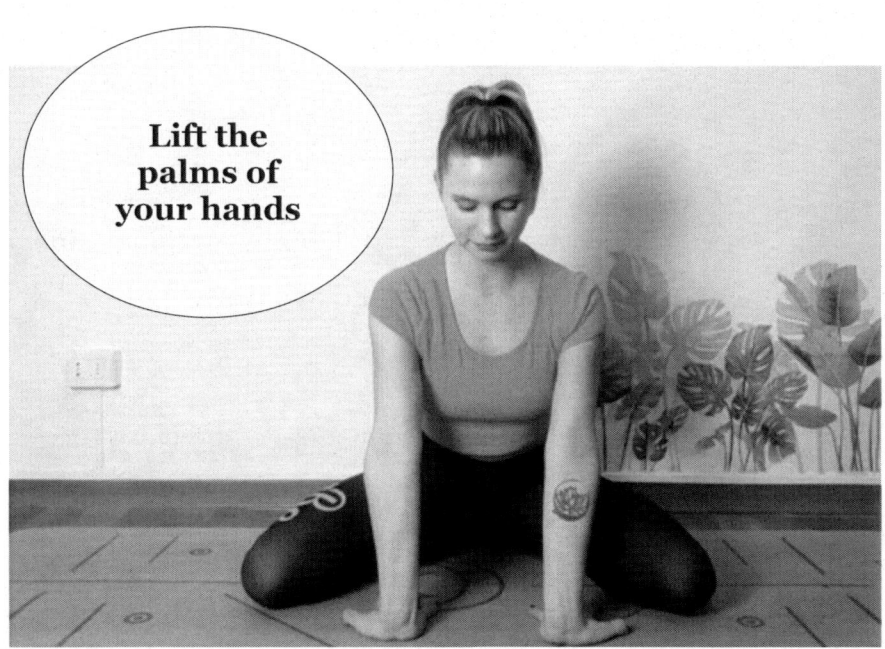

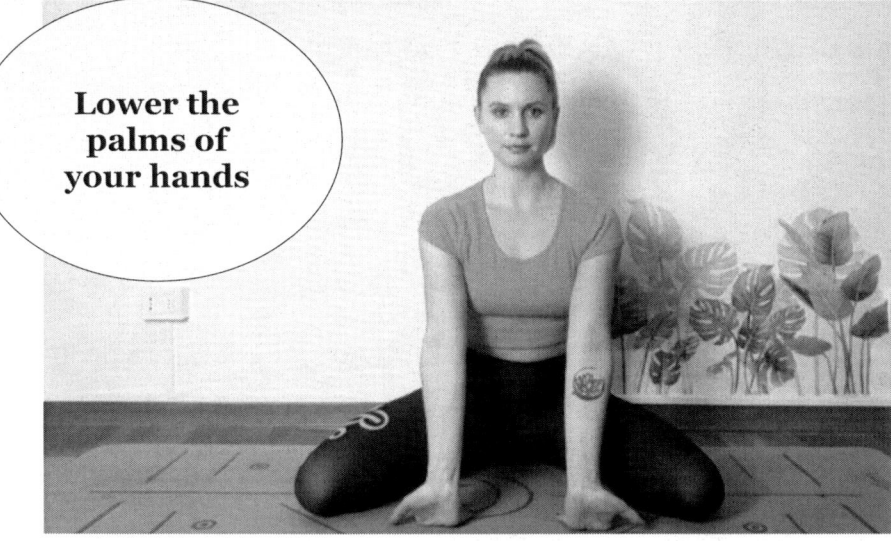

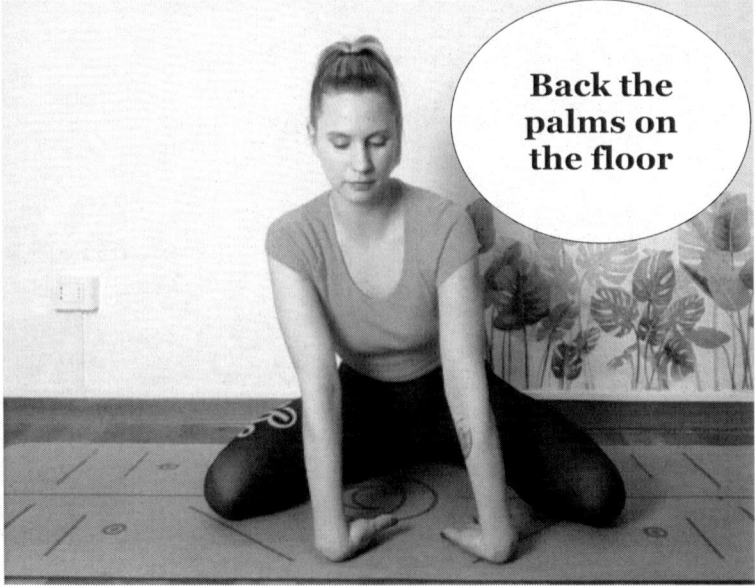

Movement Flow: Exercise 3 – Dragon

Benefits

The gentle nature of the Dragon exercise makes it very useful for recovering from injuries and reducing chronic pain. It supports the rehabilitation process and facilitates healing in the body.

Instructions

1. Go into a tabletop position: bring your left leg forward, knee in line with your ankle. Place both hands in parallel to the left foot.

2. Gently push your hips down. Hold the position for 60 seconds.

TIPS

Keep your neck long and your spine straight without rounding your back.

3. Step your left leg back and lift your hips up into a downward facing dog position, by lowering and raising your heels alternately with a slow and fluid motion.

4. Walk it out and step your right leg forward and repeat dragon pose on the opposite side. Hold the position for 60 seconds.

Breathing

Slowly brief during the exercise.

Repetitions, Sets, and Rest

Hold the Dragon position for 60 second each leg.

Suitable for

Recovering injuries and support the rehabilitation.

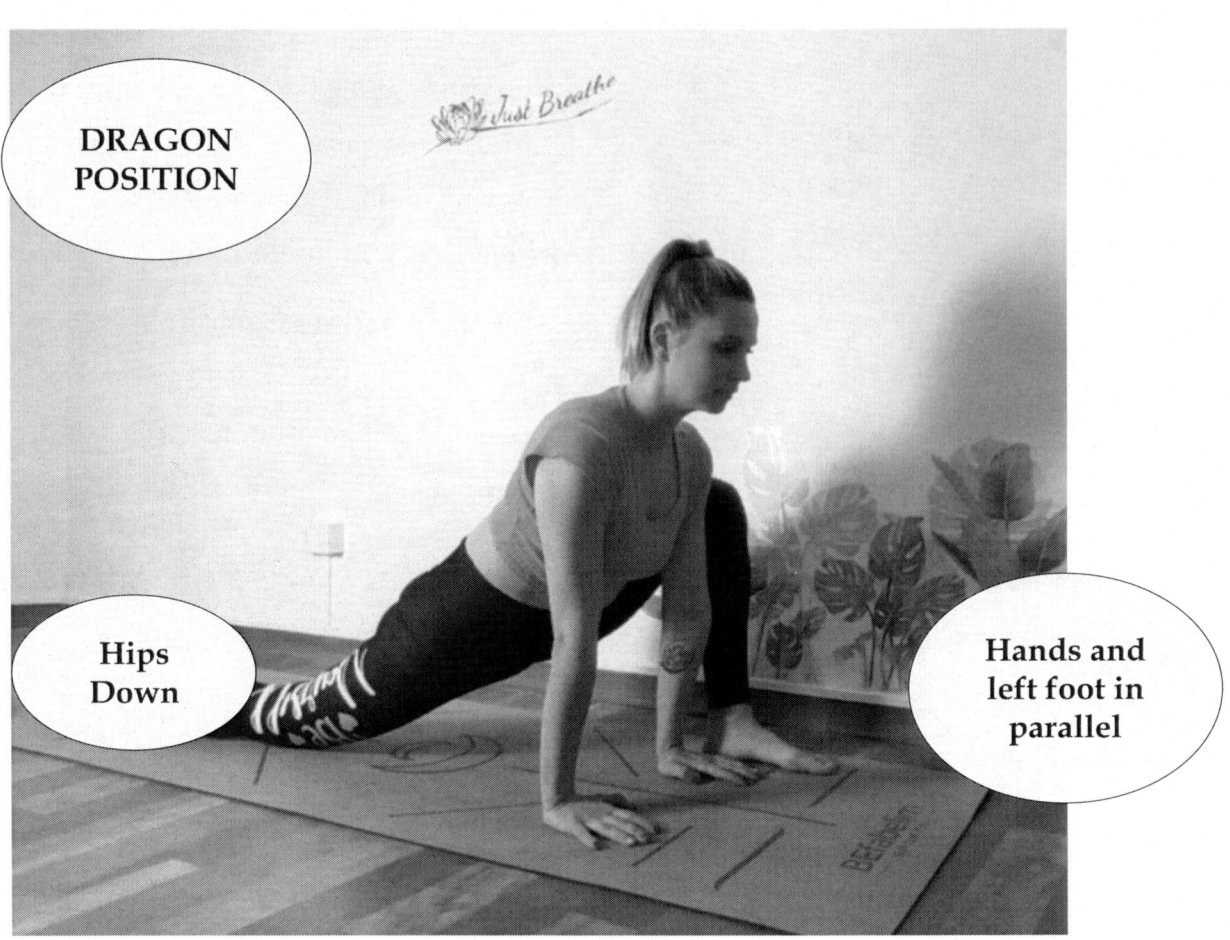

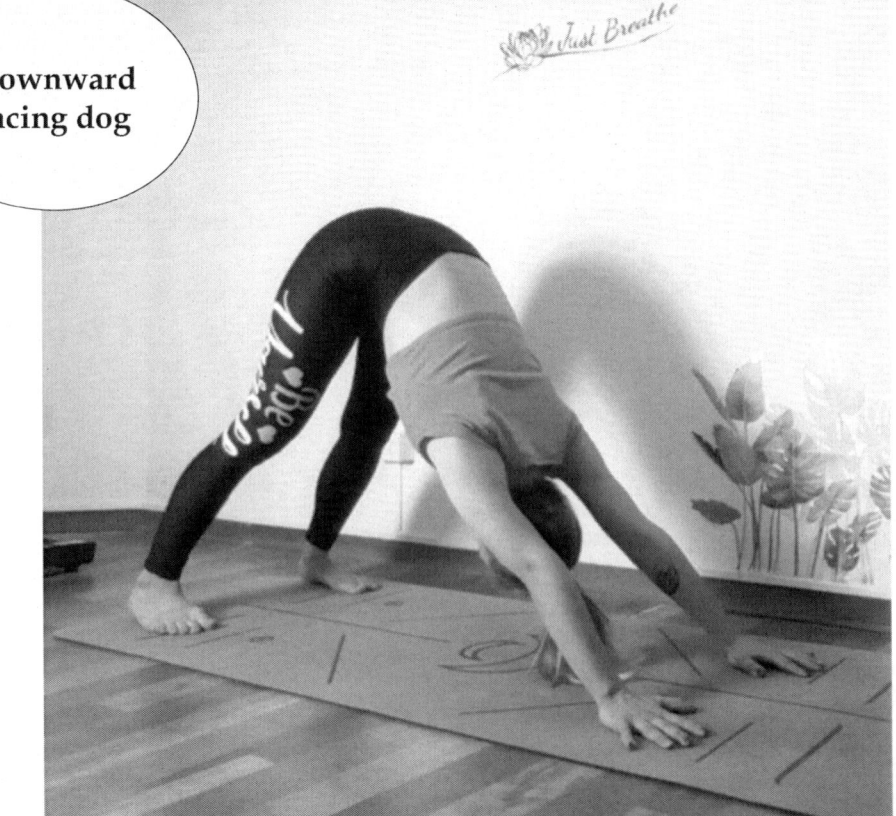

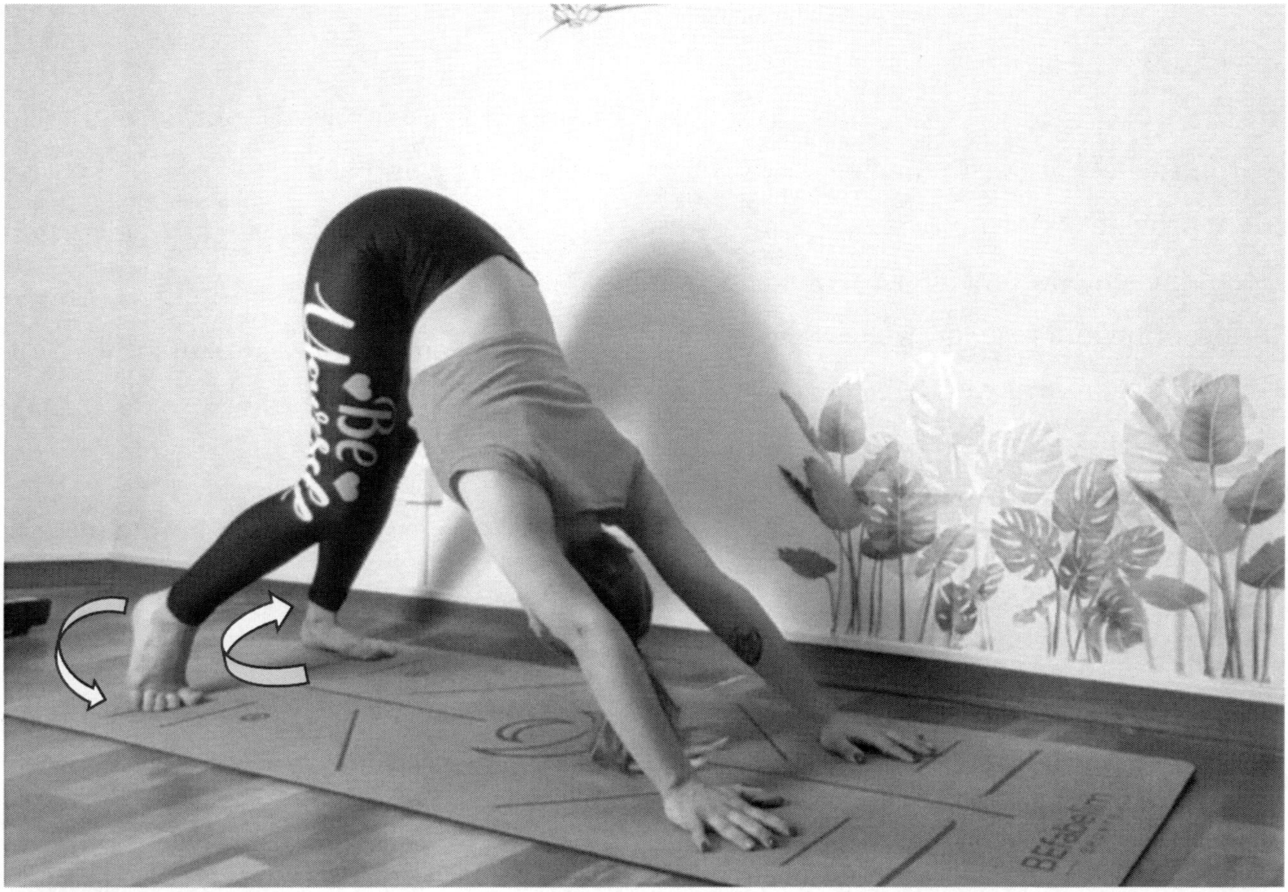

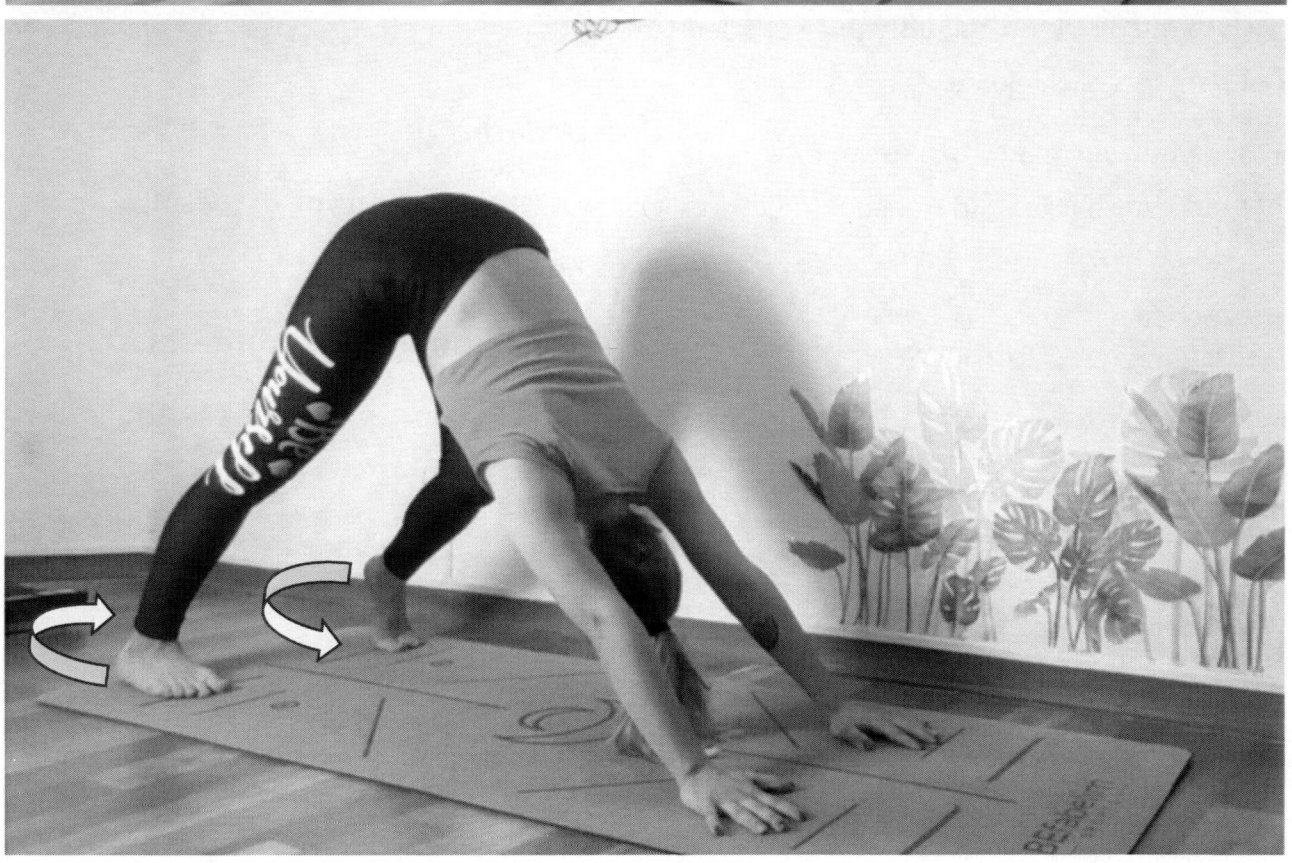

Movement Flow: Exercise 4 – Dragon Variations

Benefits

The proposed variations to the Dragon exercise provide opportunities to explore different movements and angles, enhancing proprioception and body awareness through varied and dynamic movements. Additionally, they support the exploration of different sensations and experiences within the body, fostering a deeper mind-body connection.

Instructions

1. Go into a dragon pose with your left foot forward.

2. Twist your body on the left: put your left hand on top of the knee.

3. Bring your left hand up. and then wrap it behind your back. Hold the position.

Variation 2 – Dragon stale

1. Bend the back knee, reach back and hold the foot.

TIPS

whichever variation you choose, make sure you roll the left shoulder back, your neck long and gaze upward, spine straight without rounding your back.

2. Release the left arm up and all the way back down to the ground. Lower down onto your elbows and breathe. You can always rock gently side to side. if that feels comfortable.

3. Slowly go up, bringing both hands on top of your knee, back straight. Hold the position for few seconds.

5. Go into the Downward dog position. Hold the position for few seconds. You can also lower and raise your heels alternately with a slow and fluid motion.

Breathing

Slowly breath during the exercise.

Repetitions, Sets, and Rest

Hold the position of the variation pose you chose for 2 minutes

Suitable for

enhancing proprioception and body awareness.

VARIATION
1
Just Breath

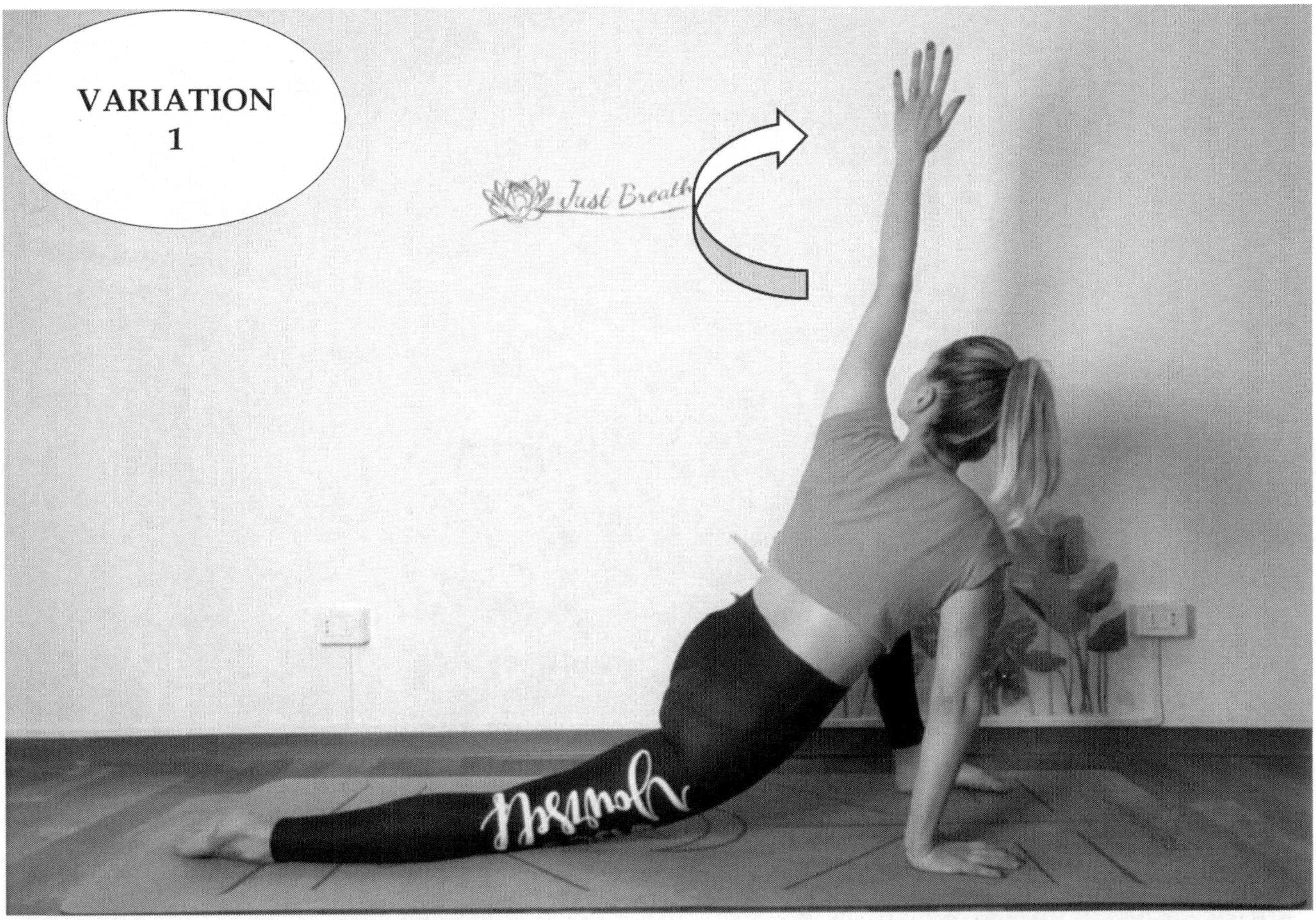

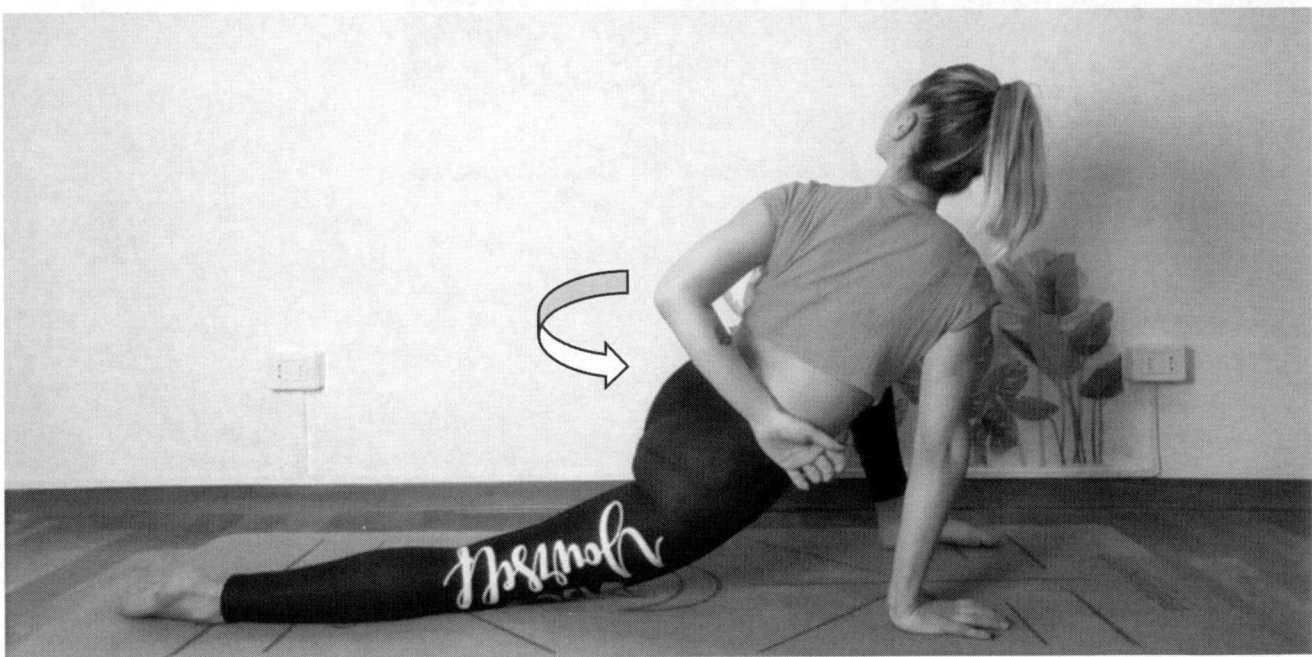

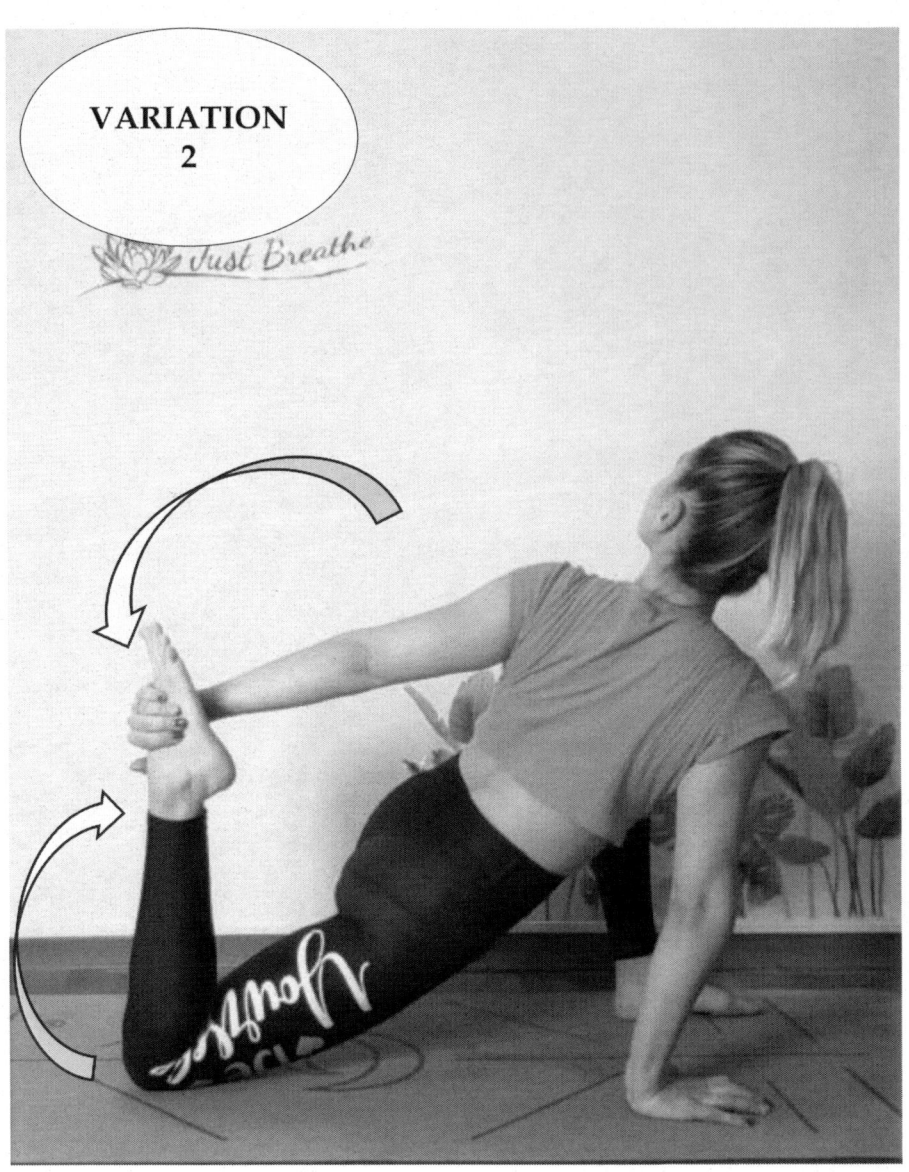

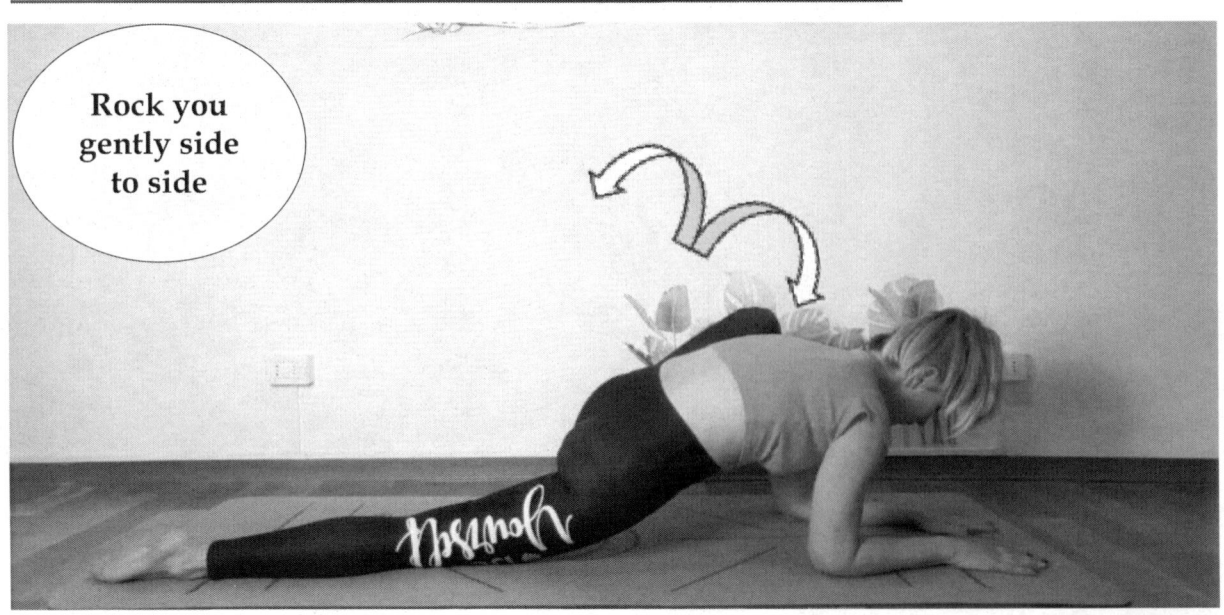

Movement Flow: Exercise 5 – Half Saddle

Benefits

The Half Saddle pose primarily targets the hip flexors, including the psoas and rectus femoris muscles. By gently stretching these muscles, it can help alleviate tension and tightness in the hips.

Instructions

1. Lie down on your back with your knees bent and your ankles in line with your knees. Bring your right knee down and let your left knee fall out to the side.

2. Hold the position and breathe deeply.

TIPS

If you want to intensify the stretch, you can bring your right foot closer to your right hip.

3. Keep your arms by your sides or raise them up above your head.

VARIATIONS

Variation 1 for intermediates

lift your left knee up.

Variation 1 for beginners

Extend your left leg on the floor.

Variation 2

Place the left foot on top of the right knee and let your knee fall down to the side.

Variation 3

Grab your left knee with your hands and pull it gently towards your chest.

Breathing

Slowly breath during the exercise.

Repetitions, Sets, and Rest

Hold the position of the variation pose you chose (Half Saddle, Variation 1, 2, or 3 you) for 2minutes.

Suitable for

Alleviate tension and tightness in the hips.

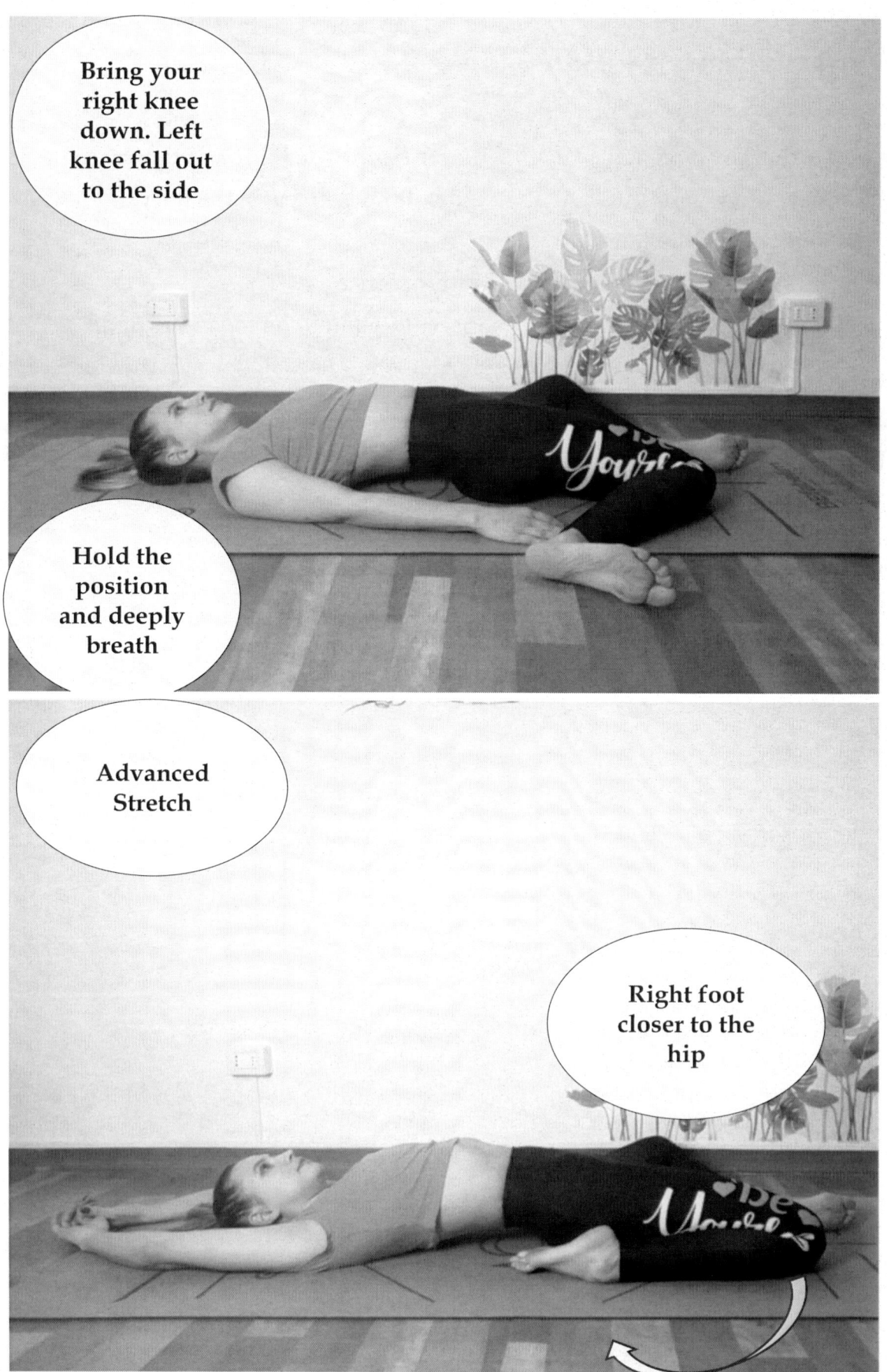

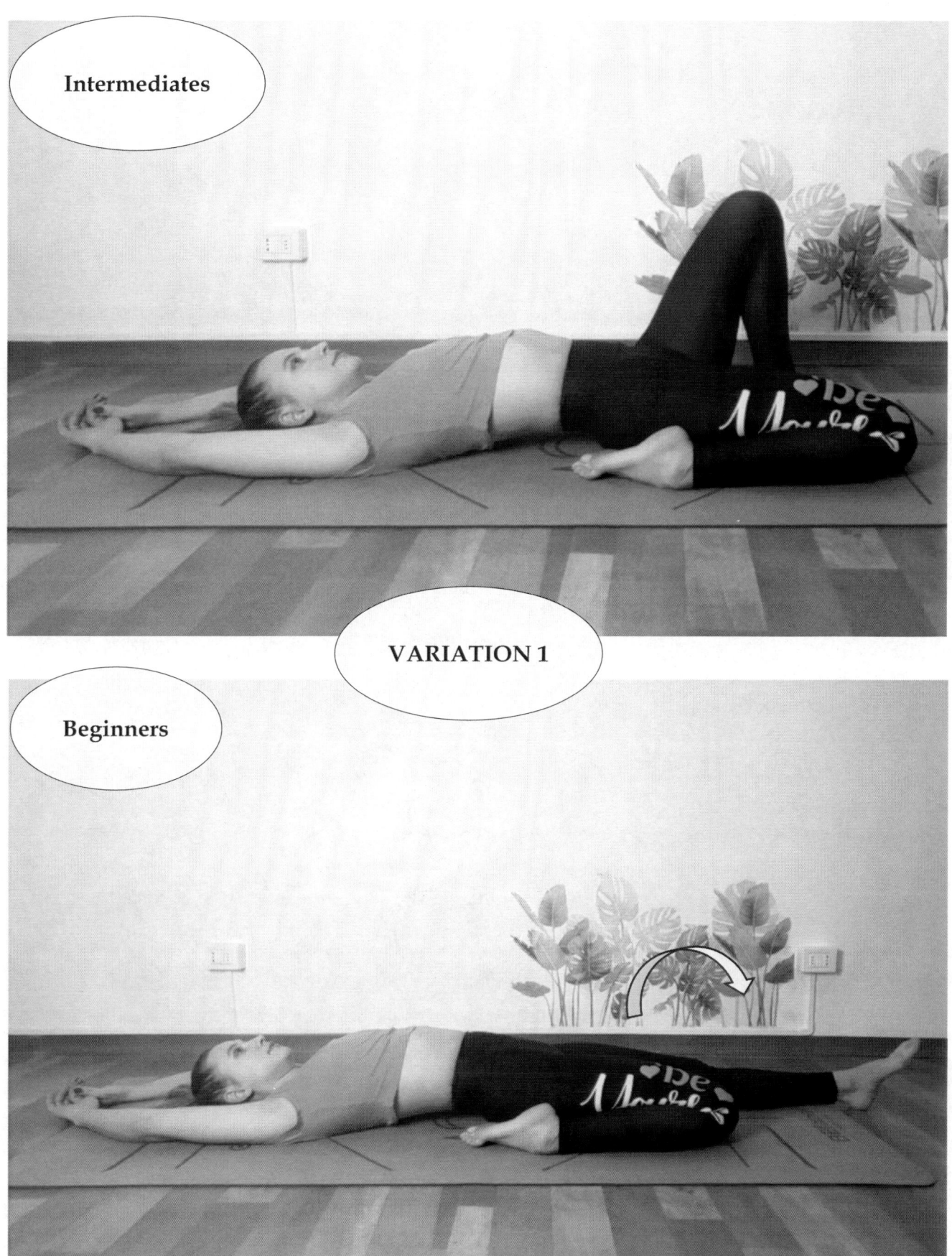

Intermediates

VARIATION 1

Beginners

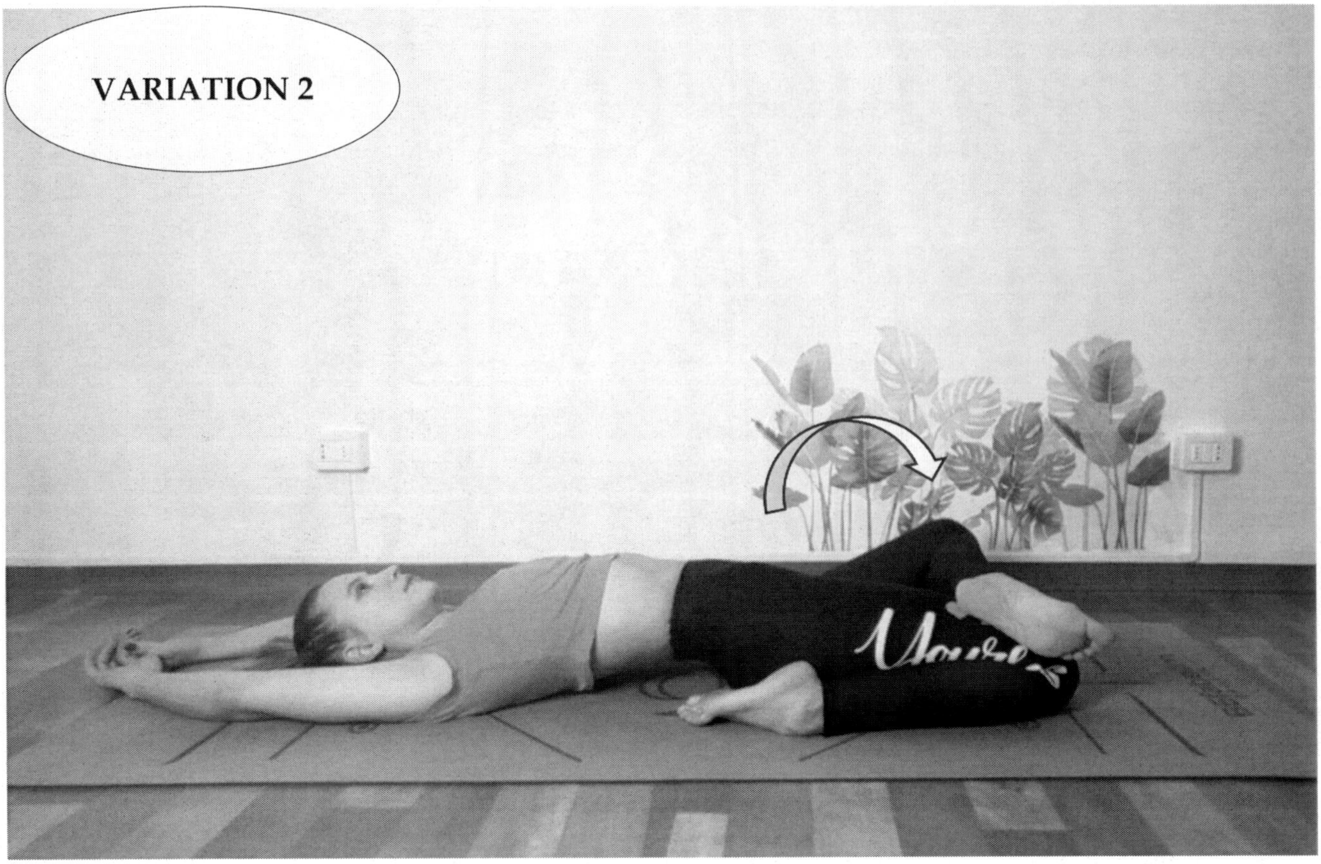

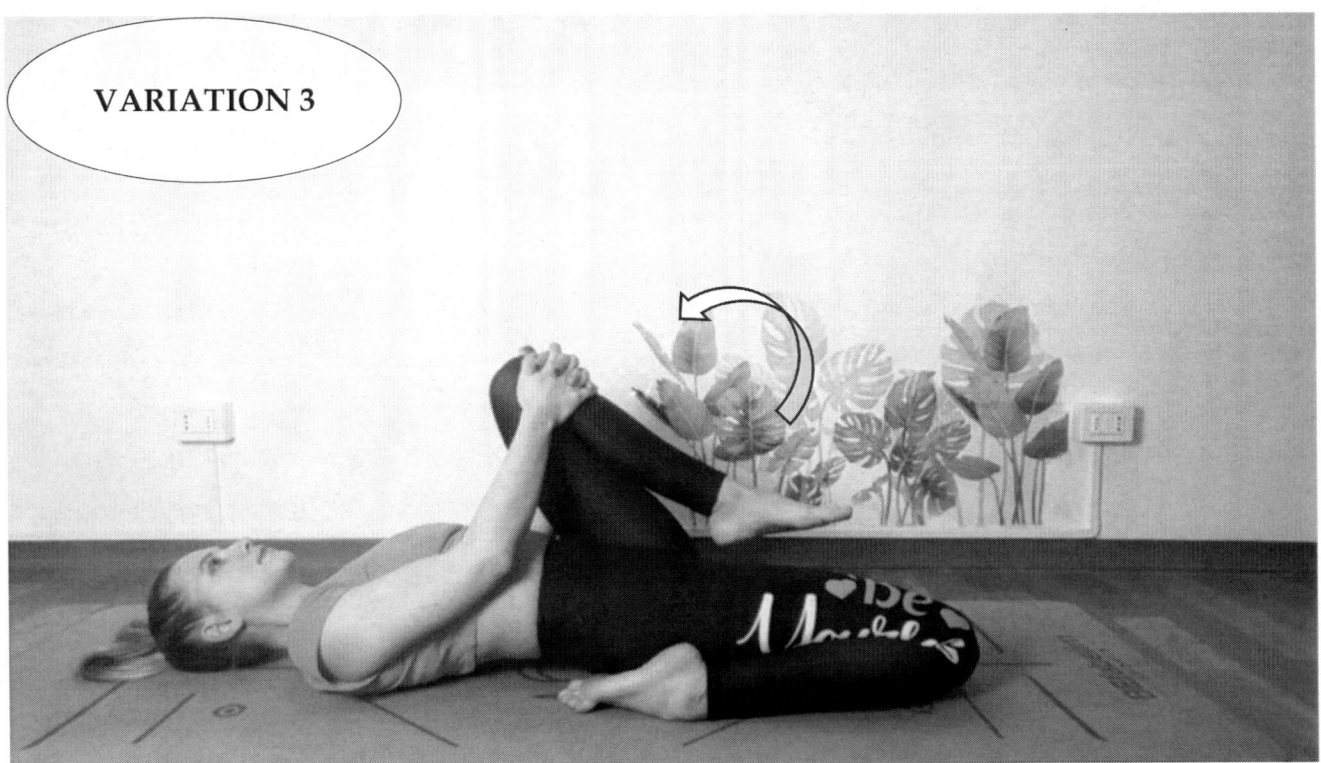

VARIATION 2

VARIATION 3

Movement Flow: Exercise 6 – Happy Baby

Benefits

The Happy Baby pose, also known as Ananda Balasana, offers various benefits: hip opening, lower back relief, stress reduction, pelvic floor activation, and Mindfulness and body awareness.

Instructions

1. Lie down on your back, arms by your sides. Bend your knees toward your chest.

2. grip the outsides of your feet with your hands. Open your knees slightly wider than your torso. Hold them your your hands.

3. Position each ankle over the knee, shins perpendicular. to the floor. Flex your feet. Gently push your feet up into your hands as you pull your hands down to create resistance.

4. Extend your spine by lengthening your tailbone and draw your belly slightly in.

Maintain the length in the back of your neck. Hold the position for 30 - 60 seconds.

TIPS

For higher benefit, gently move your knees.

Breathing

Exhale as you bend your knees to the belly, then breathe normally.

Repetitions, Sets, and Rest

5. Hold the Happy baby position for 30 - 60 seconds for 1 - 2 sets, resting 30 seconds each set.

Suitable for

Pelvic floor activation, and Mindfulness and body awareness.

**HAPPY
BABY
POSITION**

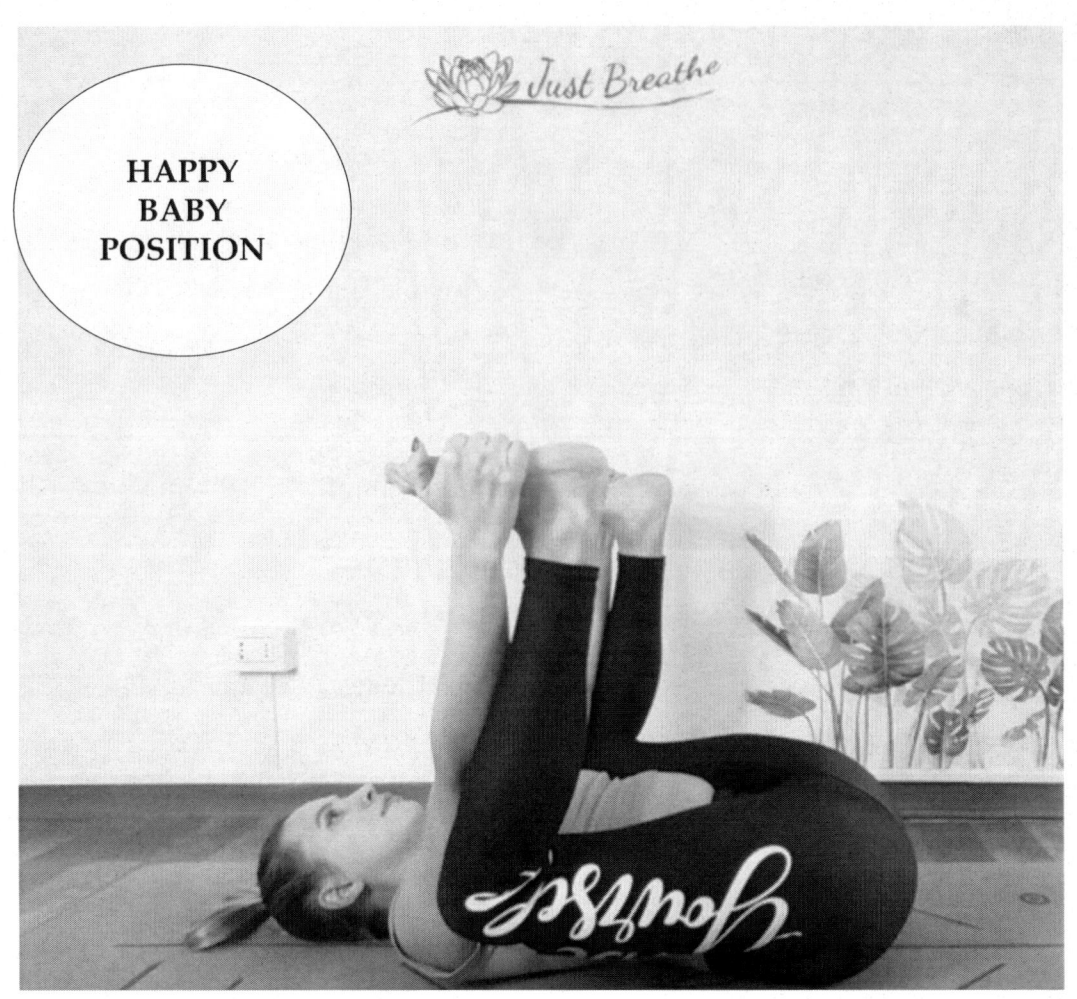

**Twist your
legs**

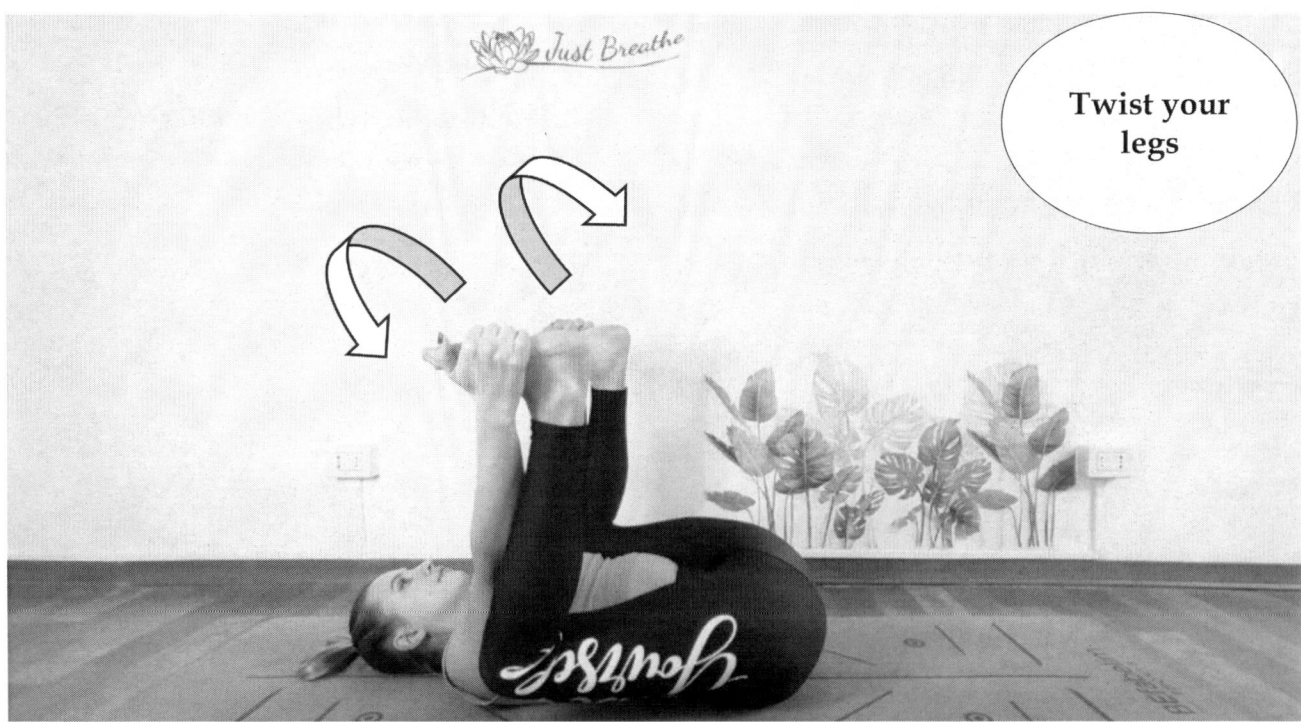

Savasana (Corpse Pose)

Benefits

This exercise implements the final relaxation pose of yoga to mindfully scan and release tension throughout the body. Bring attention to each part of the body, promoting a deep sense of relaxation.

Instructions

1. Line your back with your legs straight and arms relaxed at your sides. Let your feet fall to a natural position and rest your palms facing up.

TIP: Close your eyes. Breathe naturally. Allow your body to feel heavy on the ground.

2. Release each part of your body, organ and cell, relax your eyes, and bring attention to your breath.

3. Practice Savana for 5-10 minutes

4. Wiggle your fingers and toes, slowly reawakening your body. Stretch your arms overhead for a full body stretch.

5. Bring your knees into your chest and roll over to one side, keeping your eyes closed. Use your bottom arm as a pillow while you rest in fetal position for a few breaths.

Breathing

Breath naturally during Savana practice

Repetitions, Sets, and Rest

Practice Savasana for 5 – 10 minutes a day.

Suitable for

Promoting a deep sense of relaxation.

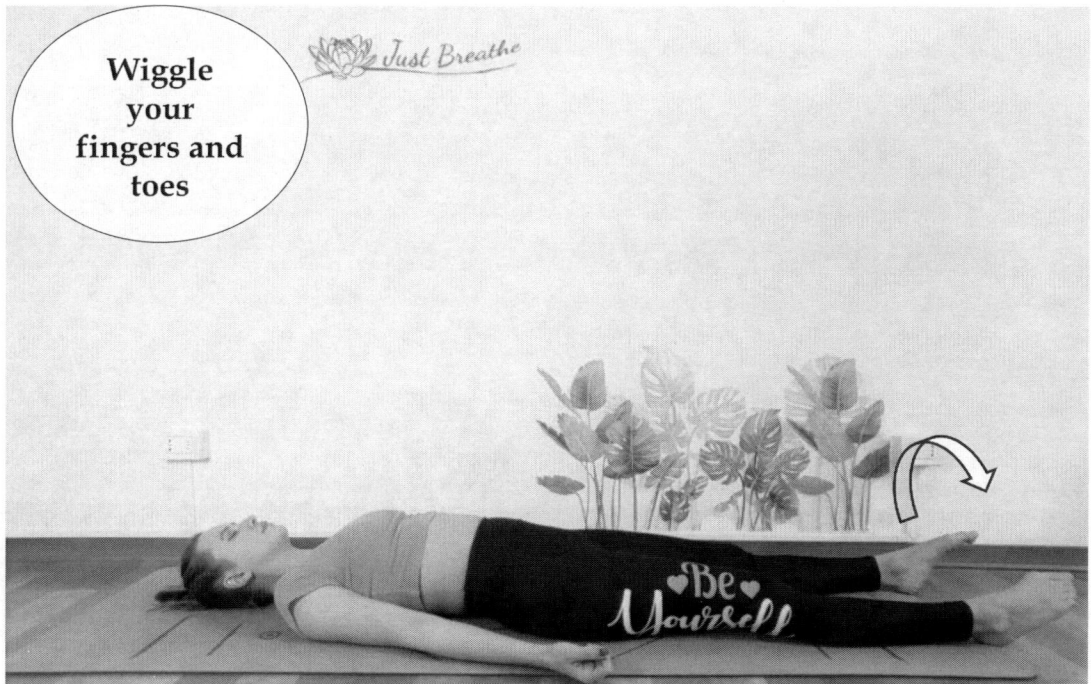

Bring your legs to your chest

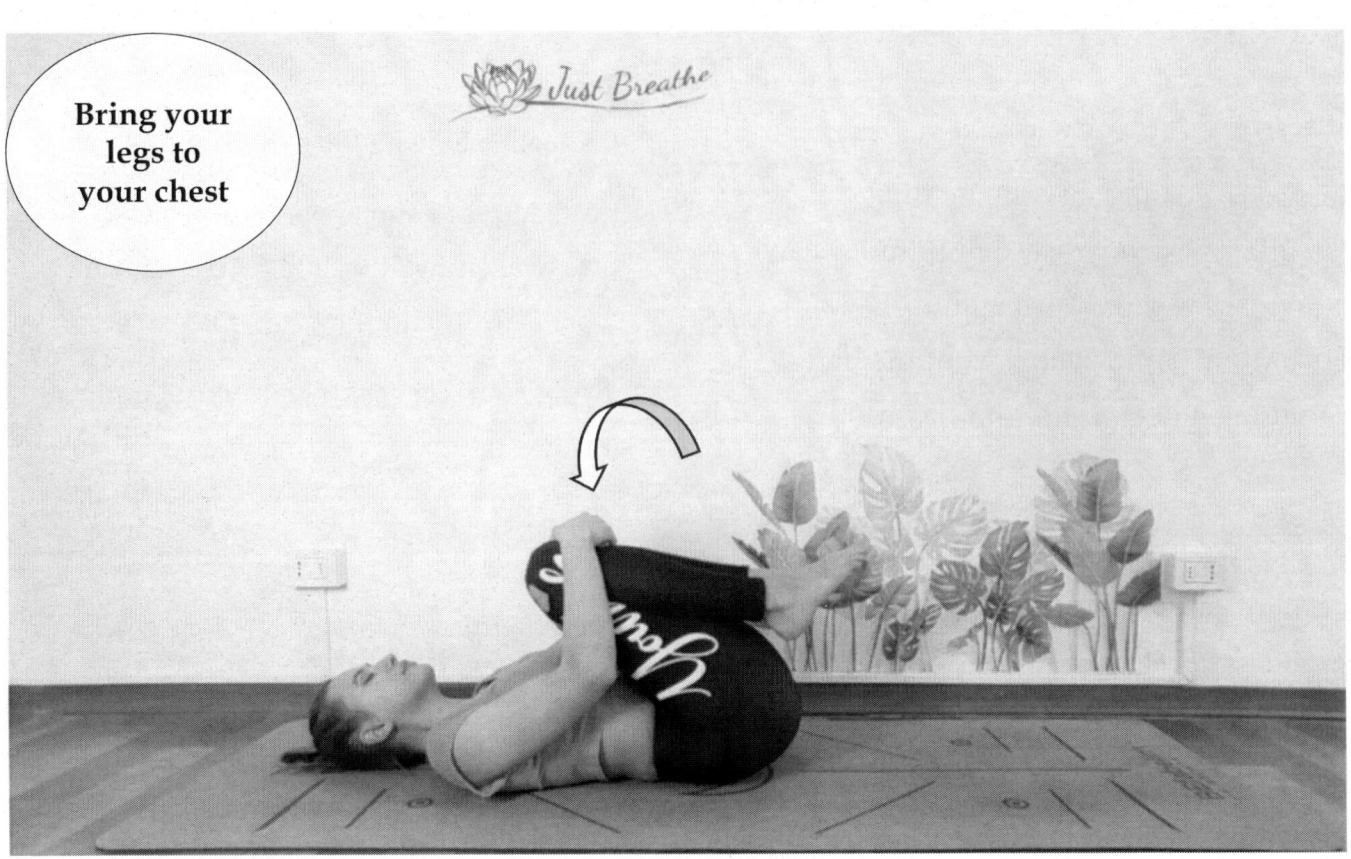

Roll over to one side

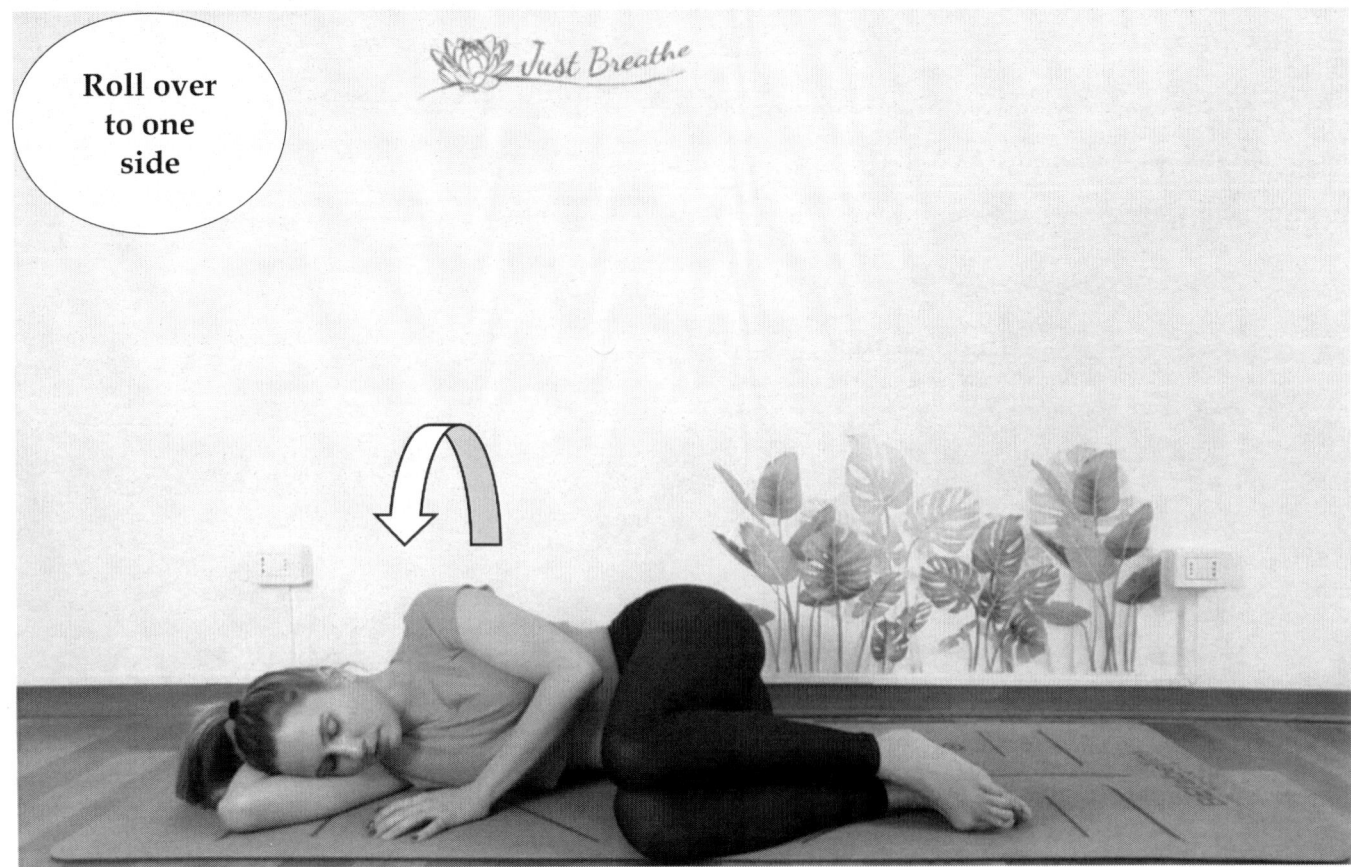

Warrior Poses

The Warrior Pose, also known as Virabhadrasana in Sanskrit, serves as a cornerstone in numerous yoga traditions, revered for its capacity to enhance strength and foster a rooted sense of being. This standing posture is celebrated for its ability to fortify and ground the practitioner.

By engaging in the Warrior Pose, you can effectively bolster the strength and flexibility of your legs, hips, and core muscles.

Furthermore, this pose facilitates the cultivation of focus, balance, and concentration, instilling a profound sense of confidence and empowerment within the practitioner.

Moreover, the Warrior Pose and its variations play a pivotal role in Somatic exercise sequences, serving as foundational postures integrated into Somatic flows and sequences to harness their several benefits.

Warrior 1 Pose

Benefits

This exercise strengthens and stretches the legs, arms, shoulders, and back. It

Improves balance and stability, opens the chest and lungs, and promotes a better breathing. It also energizes the body and mind, fostering a sense of determination and focus.

Instructions

1. Start in downward facing dog. Step the right foot forward into a lunge position, knee directly above your ankle.

2. Stand up balancing on both feet, right knee bent, left heel raised, and right foot on the floor.

3. Lower the left foot on the floor and lift your arms up, with the hands above the shoulders.

4. Hold for 30 to 60 seconds and repeat on the opposite leg.

TIPS

Press through the outer edge of the back foot. keep the chest open and shoulders down. The neck is long. Breathe.

Breathing

Inhale and raise your arms up, then exhale.

During the Warrior 1 pose normally breathe.

Repetitions, Sets, and Rest

Hold the Warrior 1 pose for 30 – 60 seconds each leg.

Suitable for

Improving balance, stability, and body energizing.

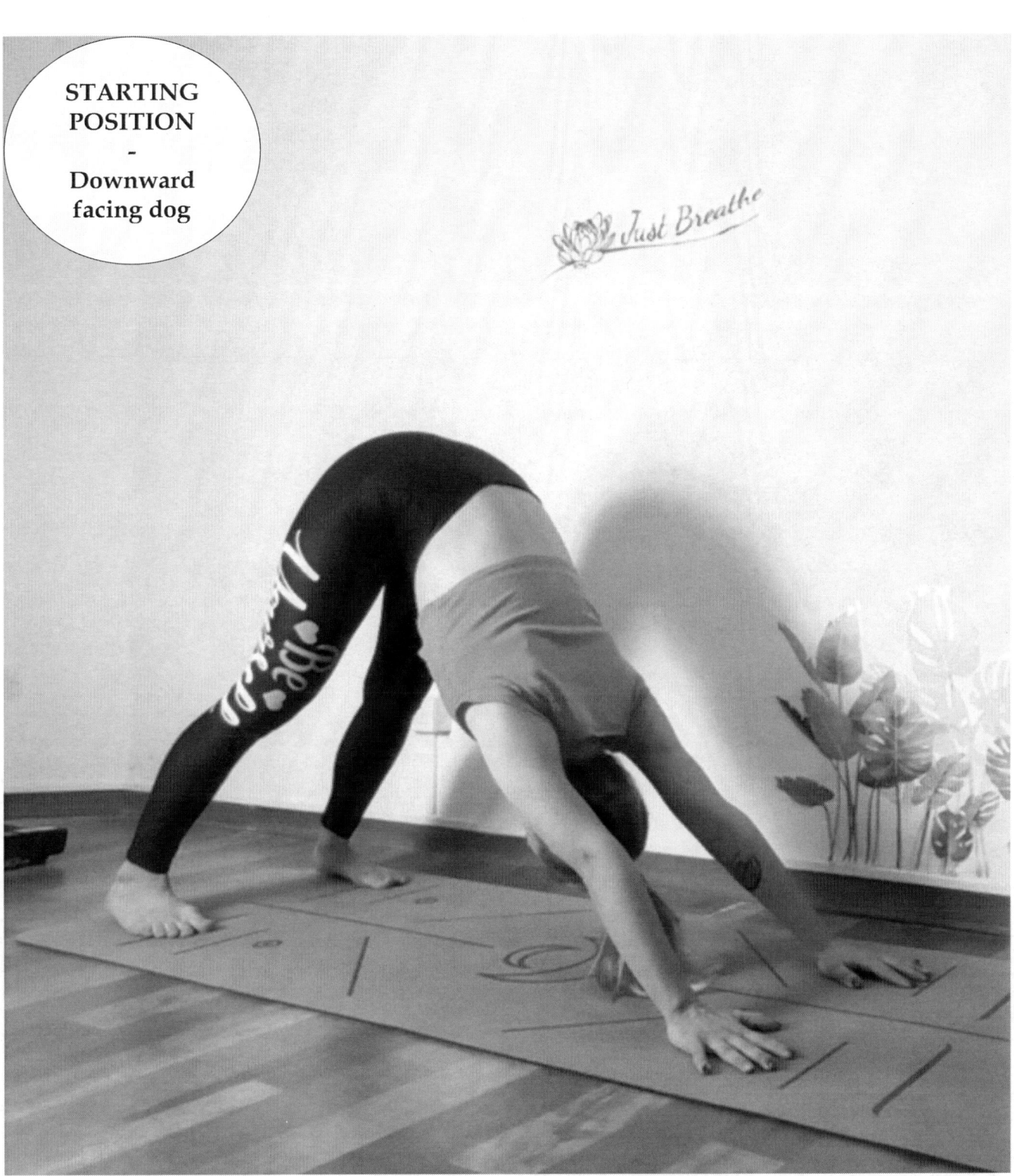

STARTING
POSITION
-
Downward
facing dog

Just Breathe

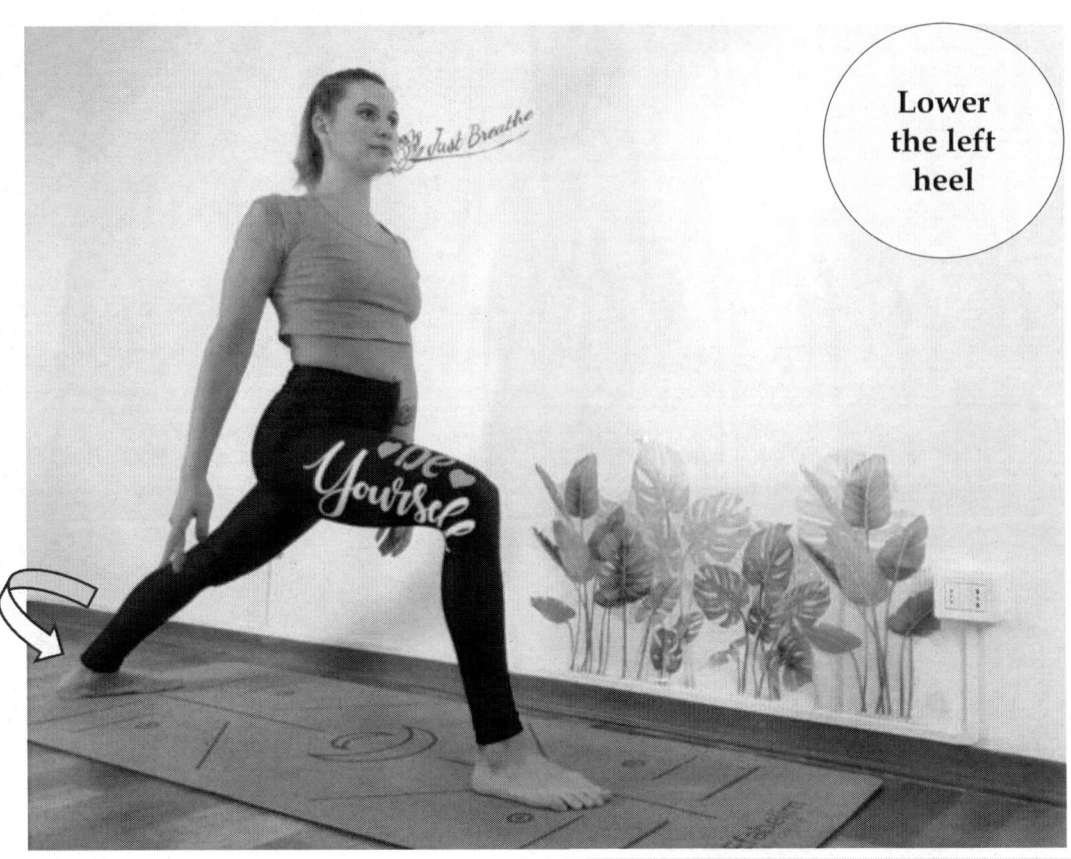

Lower
the left
heel

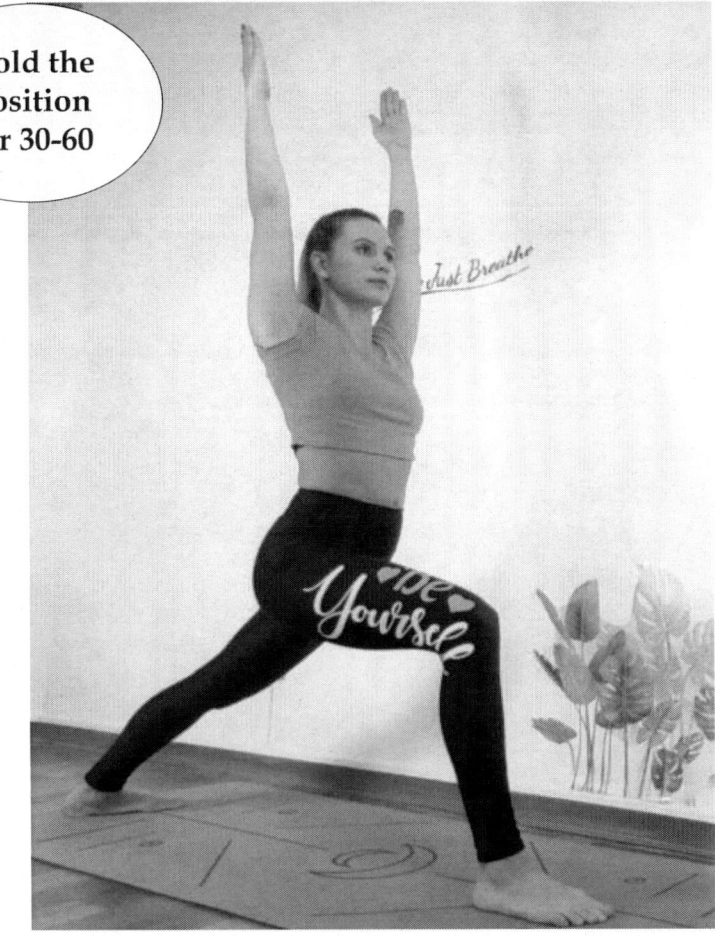

Hold the
position
for 30-60

Warrior 2 Pose

Benefits

This exercise strengthens the legs, especially the quadriceps, hamstrings, and glutes. It stretches the hips and groin area, enhancing flexibility. This pose improves concentration and mental focus as the gaze is directed forward over the front hand. It also builds stamina and endurance, both physically and mentally.

Instructions

1. Start in a downward facing dog. Step your left leg to the front of the mat. Knee at a 90-degree angle.

2. windmill your arms and extend them alongside your body, raising them parallel to the floor with your palms facing dov

3. Hold the position for 30 – 60 seconds.

4. Lift your arms, rotate your feet, and repeat the exercise with the left leg.

TIP: Keep your core gently engaged while holding the Warrior 2 position.

Breathing

Inhale as you windmill your arms.

Exhale as you lift your arms.

Repetitions, Sets, and Rest

Hold the Warrior 2 pose for 30 – 60 seconds each leg.

Suitable for

strengthening the legs, stretching the hips,

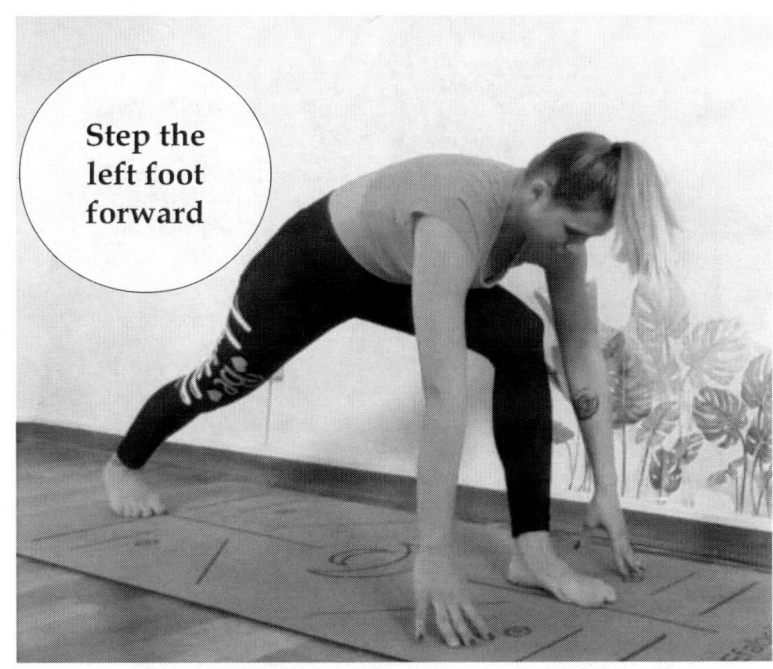

Step the left foot forward

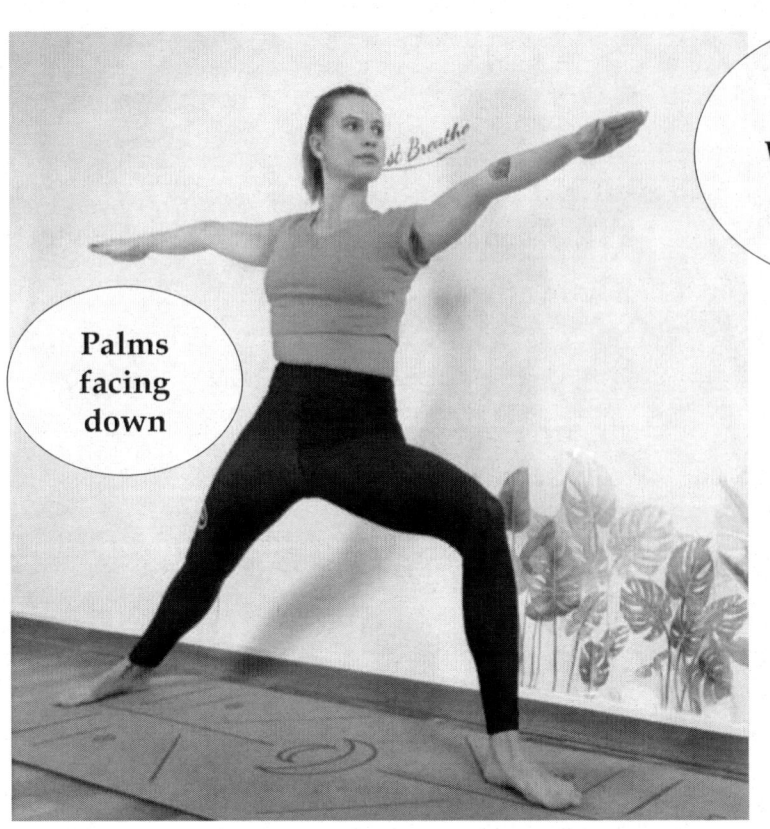

WARRIOR 2

Palms facing down

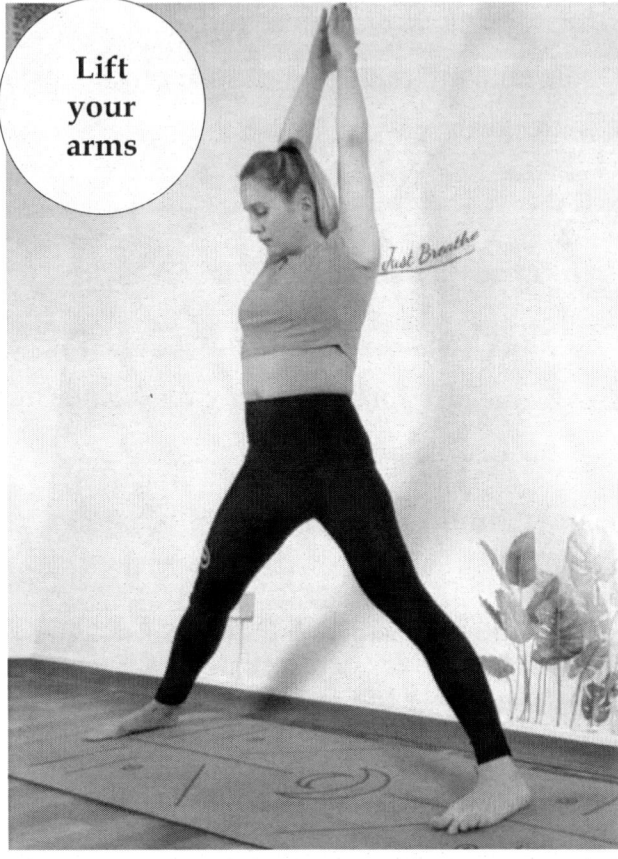

Lift your arms

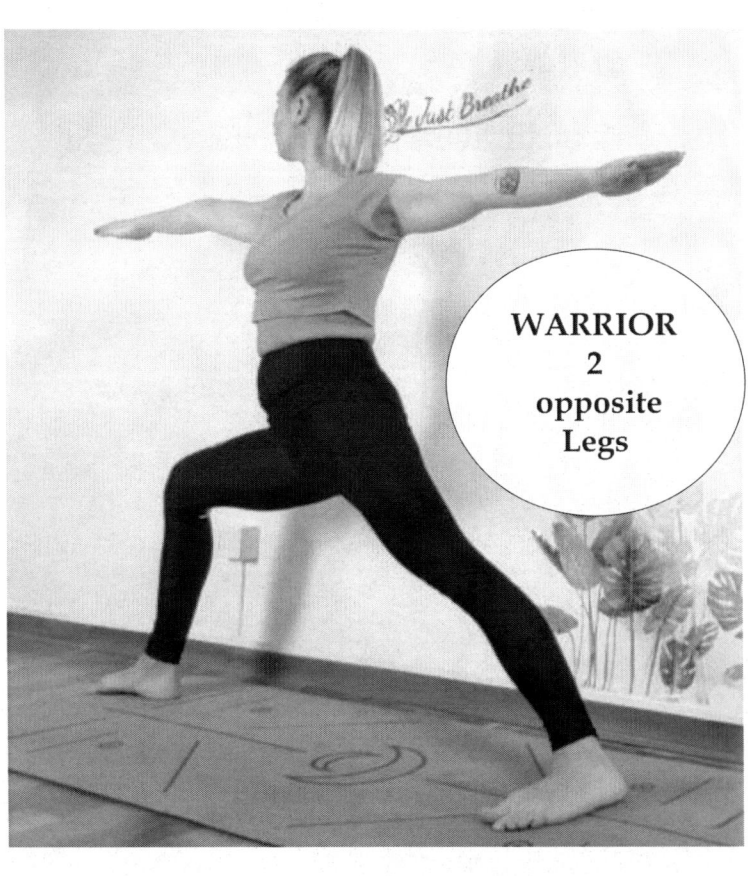

WARRIOR 2 opposite Legs

Warrior 3 Pose

Benefits

This exercise strengthens the legs, ankles, and core muscles, including the abdominals and lower back. It improves balance and coordination, as it requires alignment of the entire body in a single plane. Moreover, it cultivates mental focus and concentration, as maintaining balance in this pose requires attention and presence of mind.

Instructions

1. Begin in warrior 1 pose with your right foot forward. Your hips and chest squared to the front of the mat.

2. Move your hands to your heart with palms pressed against each other in a "prayer" position.

3. Shift your weight forward and lift your left leg out below your head.

TIP: Keep the core engaged to aid in your balance.

4. Keep your left foot flexed, square your hips and upper body down to your mat. Direct your gaze towards the floor. Try to create a "T"-shape with your body.

5. Keep your hands in a "prayer". position or extend them forward. Hold the Warrior 3 position for 30 to 60 seconds.

Breathing

Inhale as you raise your arms above your head and before shifting your weight forward.

Exhale as you move your hands to your chest and as you shift your weight forward.

Repetitions, Sets, and Rest

Hold the Warrior 3 pose for 30 – 60 seconds each leg.

Suitable for

Improving balance, coordination, and mental concentration.

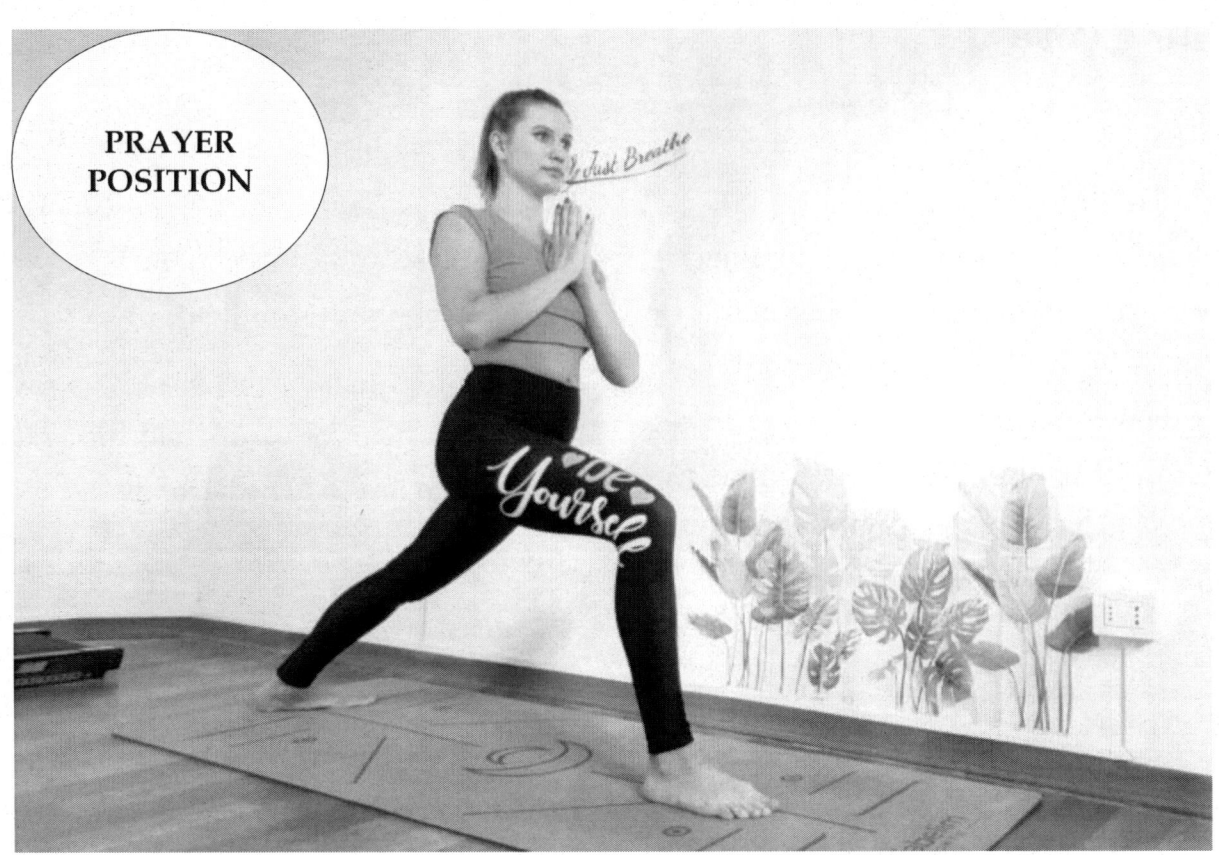

PRAYER POSITION

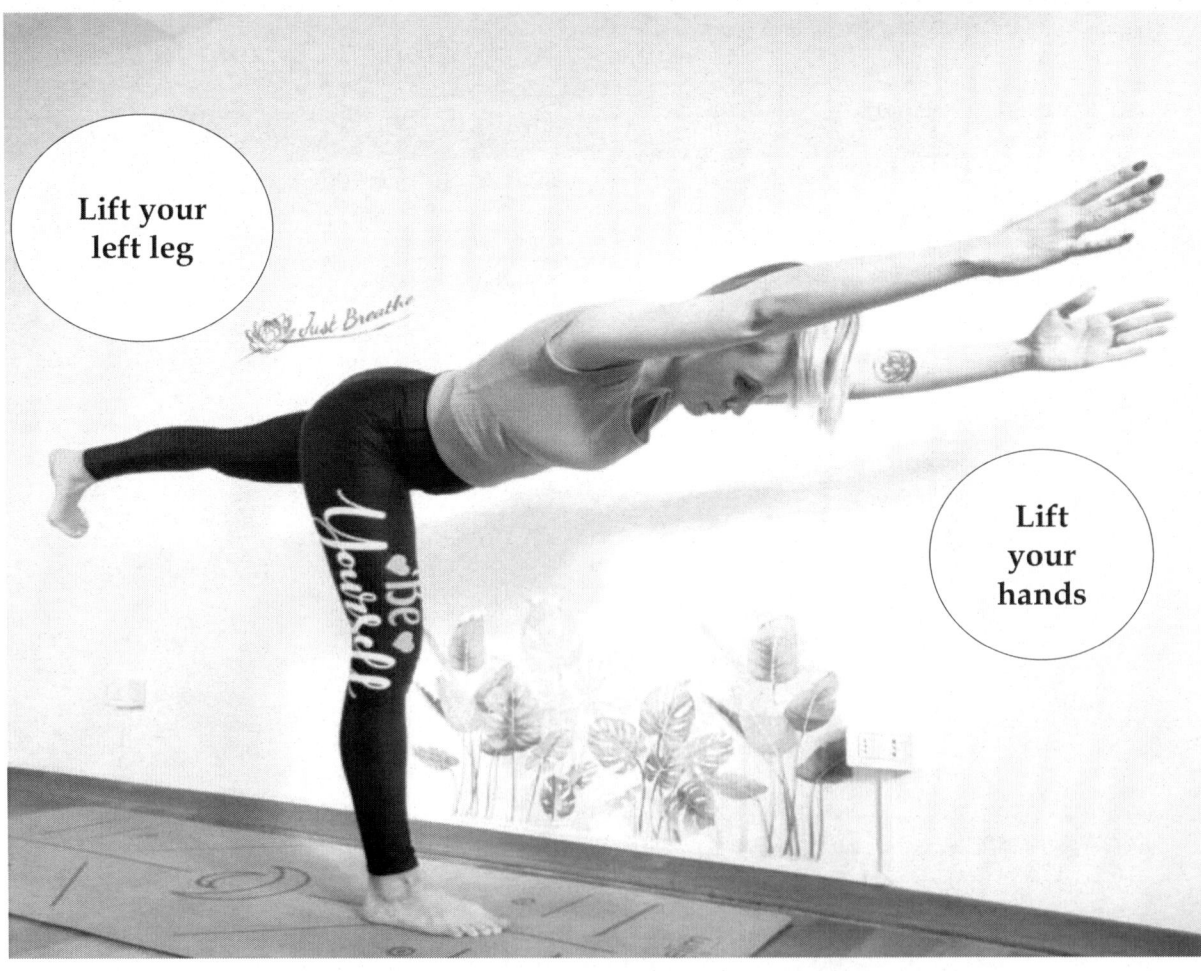

Lift your left leg

Lift your hands

Wall Pose: Legs-Up

Benefits

This exercise releases tension in the hips, lower back, and legs. Mindfully move your legs and pelvis to find areas of tightness and allow for a gentle release.

Instructions

1. Lie flat on the back and place your hips against the wall or slightly away. Place your arms in any comfortable position.

Close your eyes and relax. Breathe naturally. Stay in this position from 2 to 20 minutes.

Breathing

Breath naturally during the exercise.

Repetitions, Sets, and Rest

Hold the position for 2 – 20 minutes.

Suitable for

Release tension in the hips, lower back and legs.

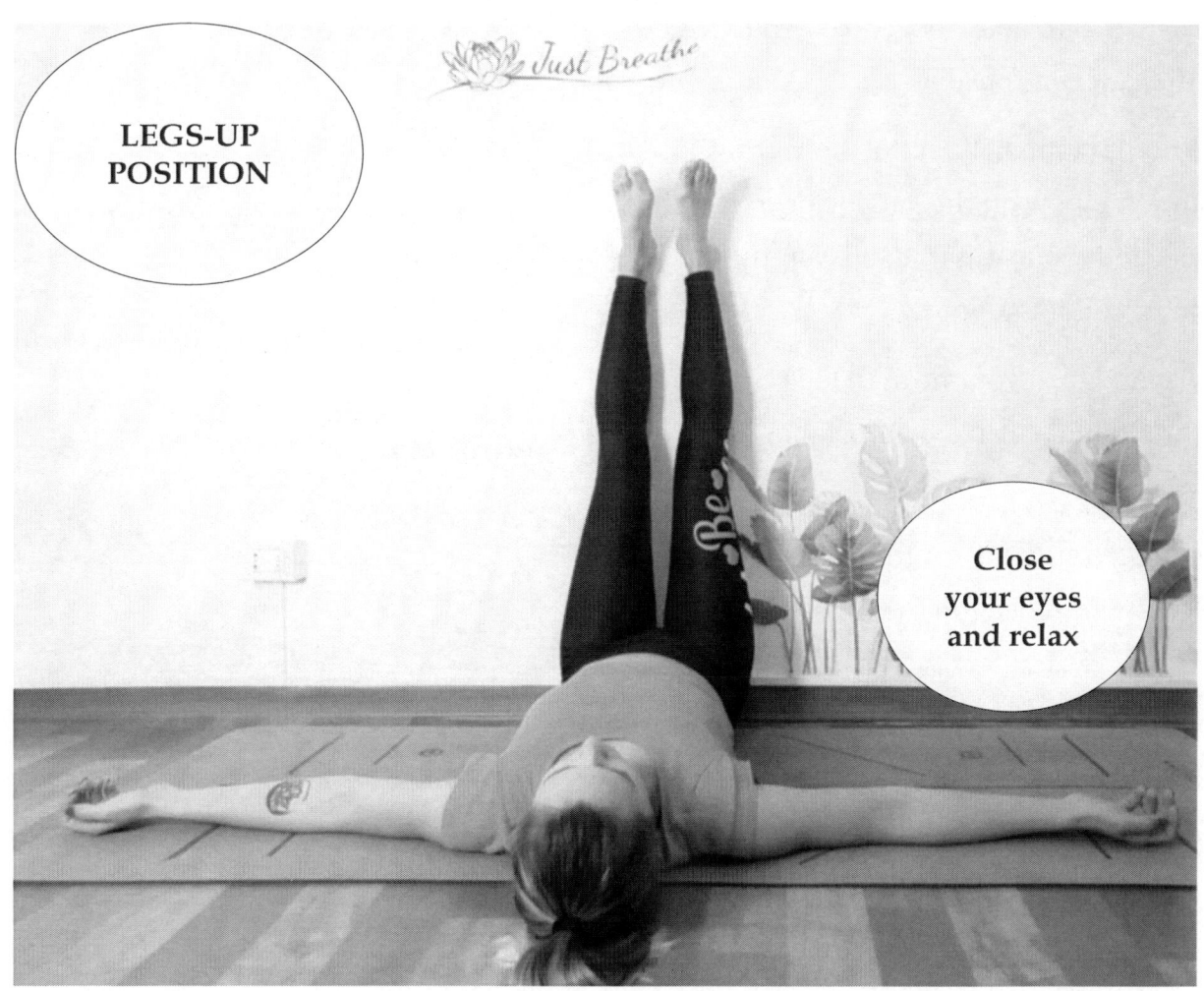

LEGS-UP POSITION

Just Breathe

Close your eyes and relax

Tower Twist

Benefits

This exercise helps release tension in the spine and promotes greater mobility.

Instructions

1. Sit on the floor with your legs extended in front of you. Keep your back straight and your shoulders relaxed.

2. Bend your right knee and place your right foot on the outside of your left knee.

3. keep your left leg straight or you can bend it with your left foot near your right buttock, if comfortable.

4. Turn your upper body to the right. Place your left elbow on the outside of your right knee and your right hand on the floor behind you for support.

5. Twist and turn your head to look over your right shoulder if it's comfortable for your neck.

6. Hold the twist for 20 to 30 seconds then release and repeat on the other side.

TIPS

keep your spine straight and elongated during the twist and avoid slouching or rounding your back. Do not force your body into a deeper twist than is comfortable.

Breathing

Inhale deeply as you sit up tall.

Exhale as you twist.

During the tower twist position keep your breathing steady and deep.

Repetitions, Sets, and Rest

Hold the twist for 20 − 30 seconds for 1 − 2 sets, resting 30 − 60 seconds each set.

Suitable for

Release the tension in your spine.

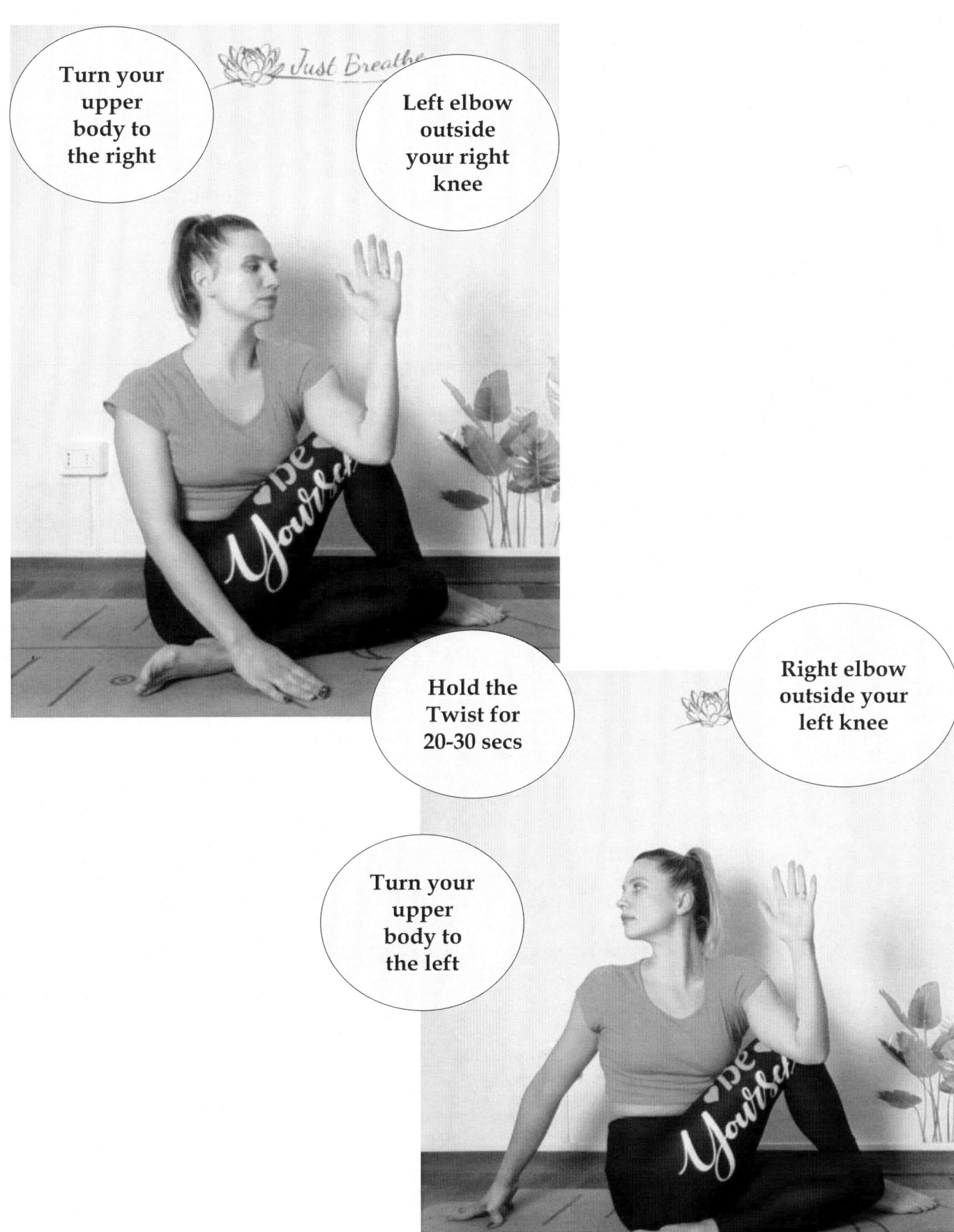

Shoulder Rolls

Benefits

This exercise helps release tension in the spine and promotes greater mobility.

Instructions

1. Stand or sit comfortably with your legs crossed. Slowly roll your shoulders in a circular motion

TIP

Pay attention to the connection between your breath and the movement, release the tension in the neck and shoulders.

2. Squeeze the shoulders up towards the ears.

3. Roll the shoulders back bringing your shoulder blades together, getting into every corner of your shoulders.

Breathing

Breathe slowly during the exercise.

Repetitions, Sets, and Rest

Reps: 5 – 10 shoulder circular rolls forward and backward.

Suitable for

Release shoulders and spine tension.

Just Breathe

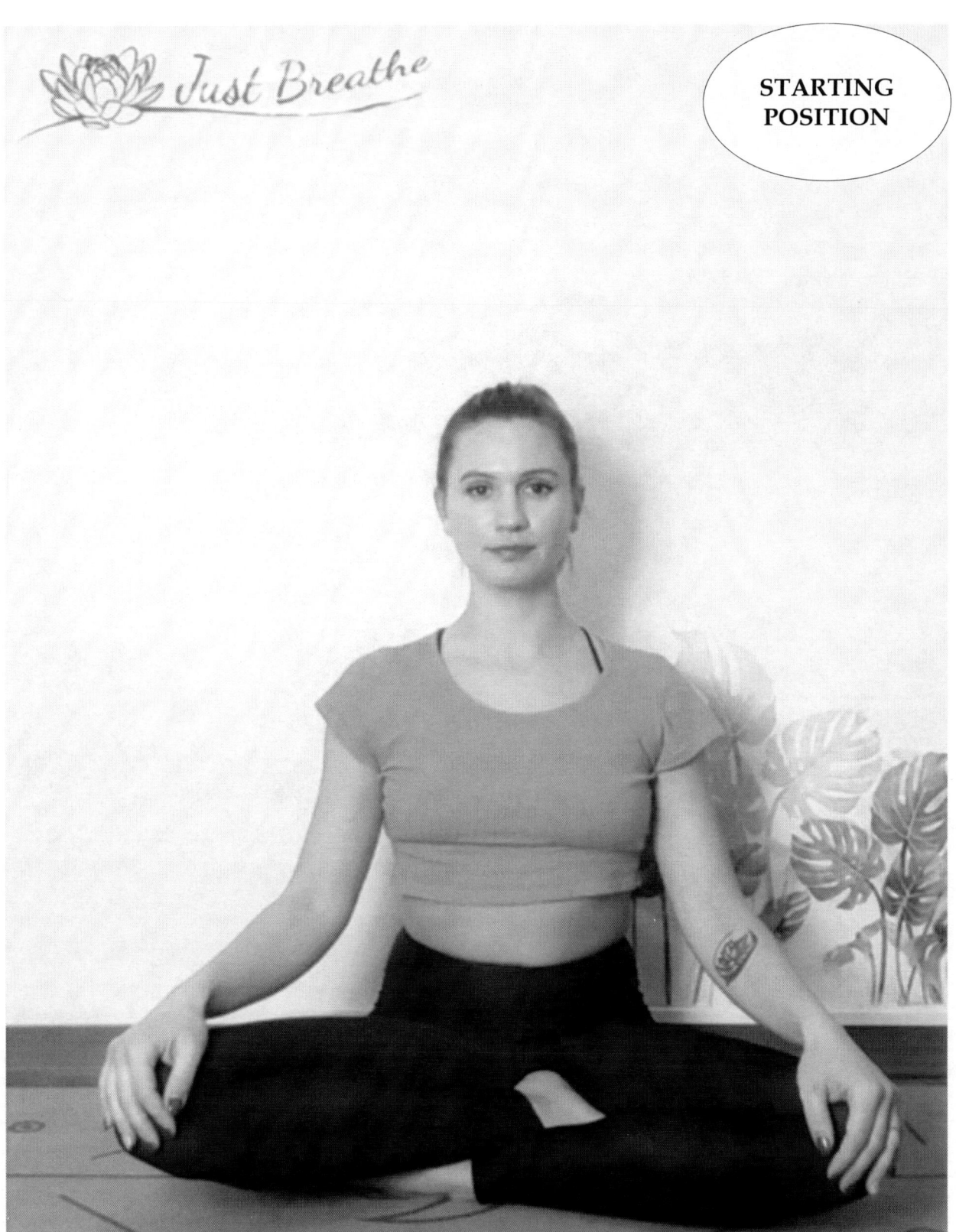

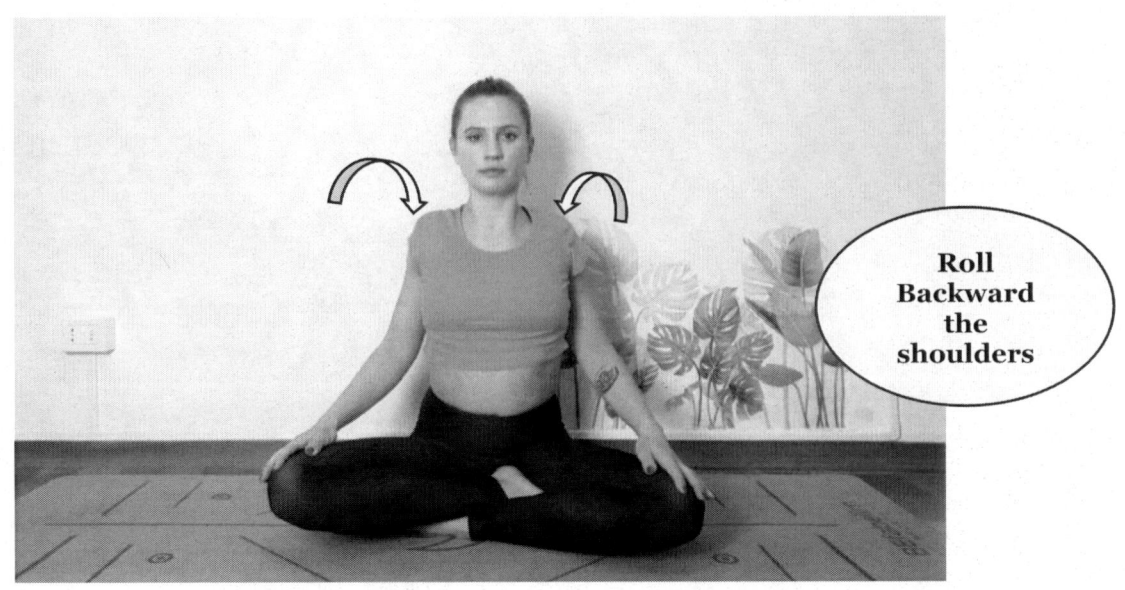

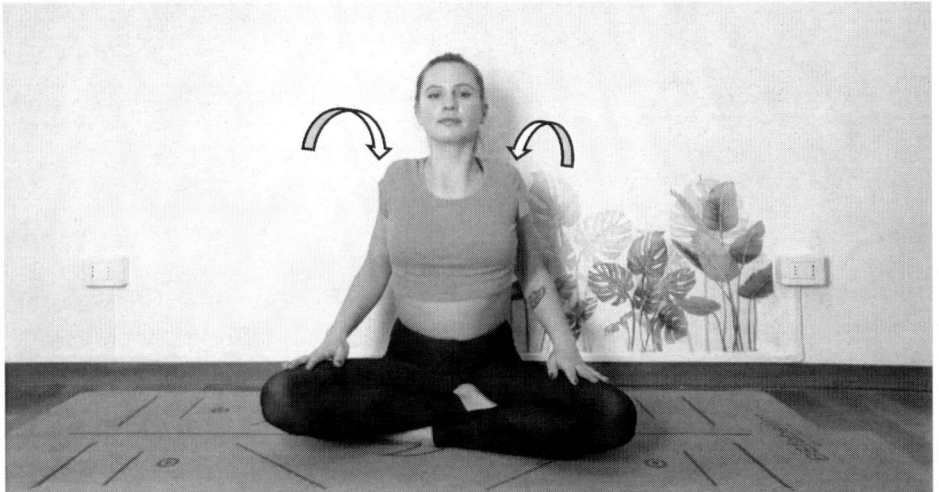

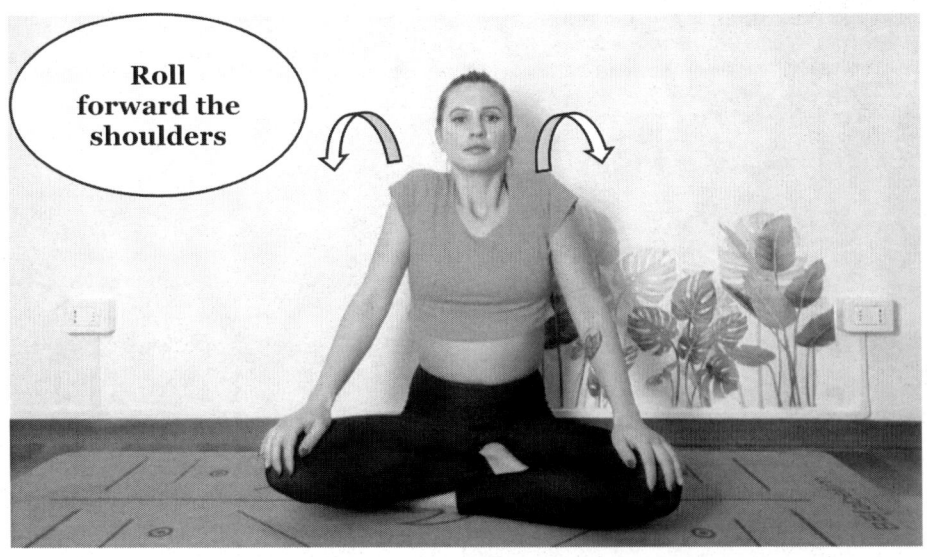

Forward Stretch of the Spine (Sagittal Plane)

Benefits

This exercise is excellent for improving Spinal flexibility and Posture. It activates Core and enhances the Body awareness.

Instructions

1. Extend legs in front, slightly wider than mat width, and toes pointing upward.

2. Lift arms to shoulder height, inhale to prepare, then exhale, curl chin to chest, reaching forward.

3. Maintain a straight spine without a "C"-curve, feeling sit bones on the mat.

TIP: For comfort, if sitting straight is difficult, bend knees slightly, lift arms, and perform the exercise.

Breathing

Inhale before initiating the movement. Exhale while performing the flexion of the spine.

Repetitions, Sets, and Rest

5 – 10 repetitions for 1 – 2 sets, resting for 30 – 60 seconds between each set.

Suitable for

Core and enhancing activation.

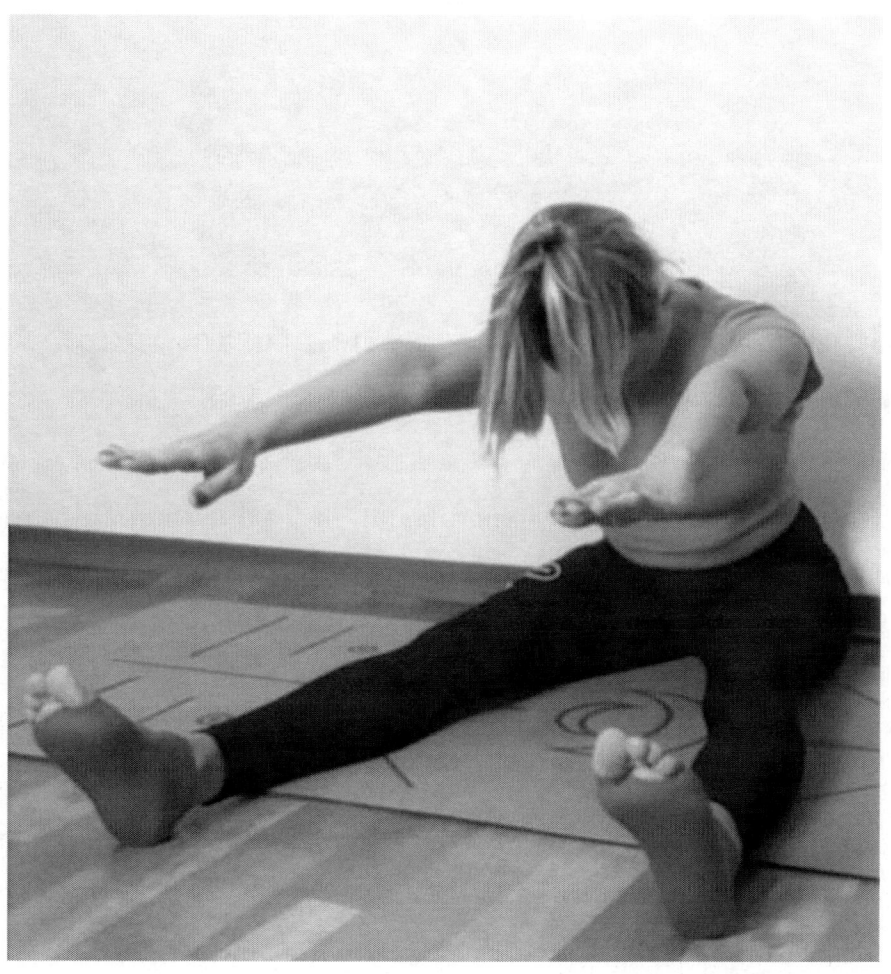

Chapter 6: Somatic Emotional Exercises

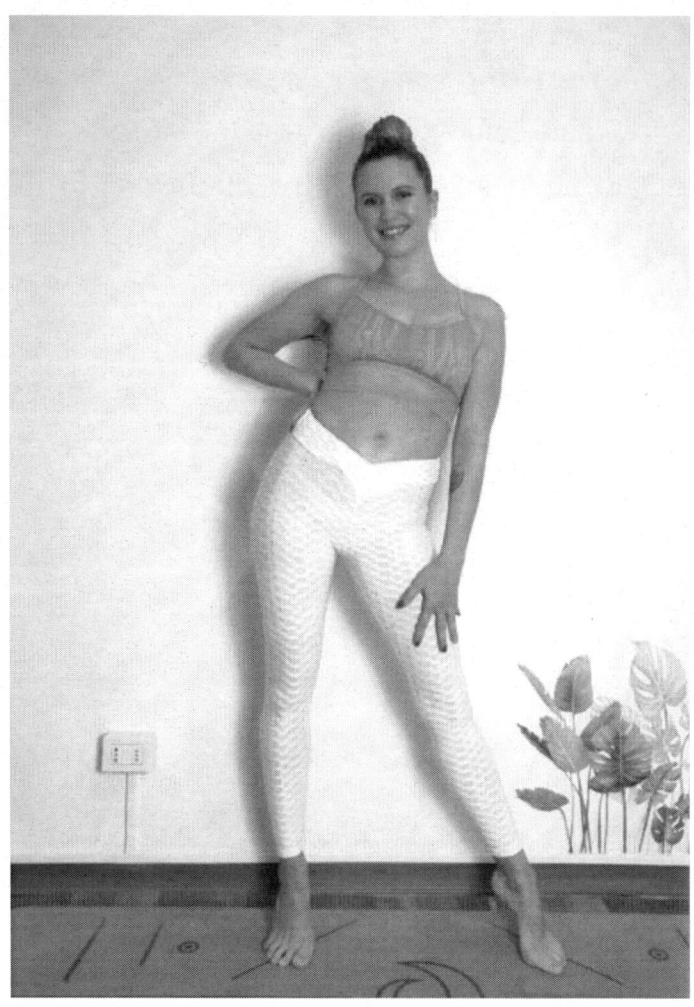

Somatic exercises are very helpful for managing difficult emotions and releasing positive emotions.

By addressing the physical manifestations of those emotions in the body, through routine practice of somatic emotional exercises, you'll become more aware of your body's responses to difficult emotions and develop healthier ways of coping with them.

Moreover, these somatic emotional exercises will help you "bring out" positive sensations, which are often too suppressed and kept inside.

In fact, these particular somatic exercises offer a unique approach to emotional well-being by focusing on the connection between the body and the mind, helping you to cultivate greater awareness, regulation, and empowerment in your life.

Release unprocessed emotions

Benefits

This exercise helps individuals to access and release emotions stored in the body, which might be otherwise difficult to express verbally. This release leads to a sense of emotional relief and catharsis.

Instructions

1. Lie down on your back with a pillow under your lower back, upper back and head. Knees bent and hip width apart.

2. Open up your arms to the sides, palms facing up. Close your eyes, breathe naturally and hold the position for 3 -5 minutes allowing your body to feel heavy and your stomach to relax.

3. Get up very slowly to finish up.

Breathing

Breath naturally during the exercise.

Repetitions, Sets, and Rest

Hold the position for 3 – 5 minutes.

Suitable for

Leading to emotional relief and catharsis

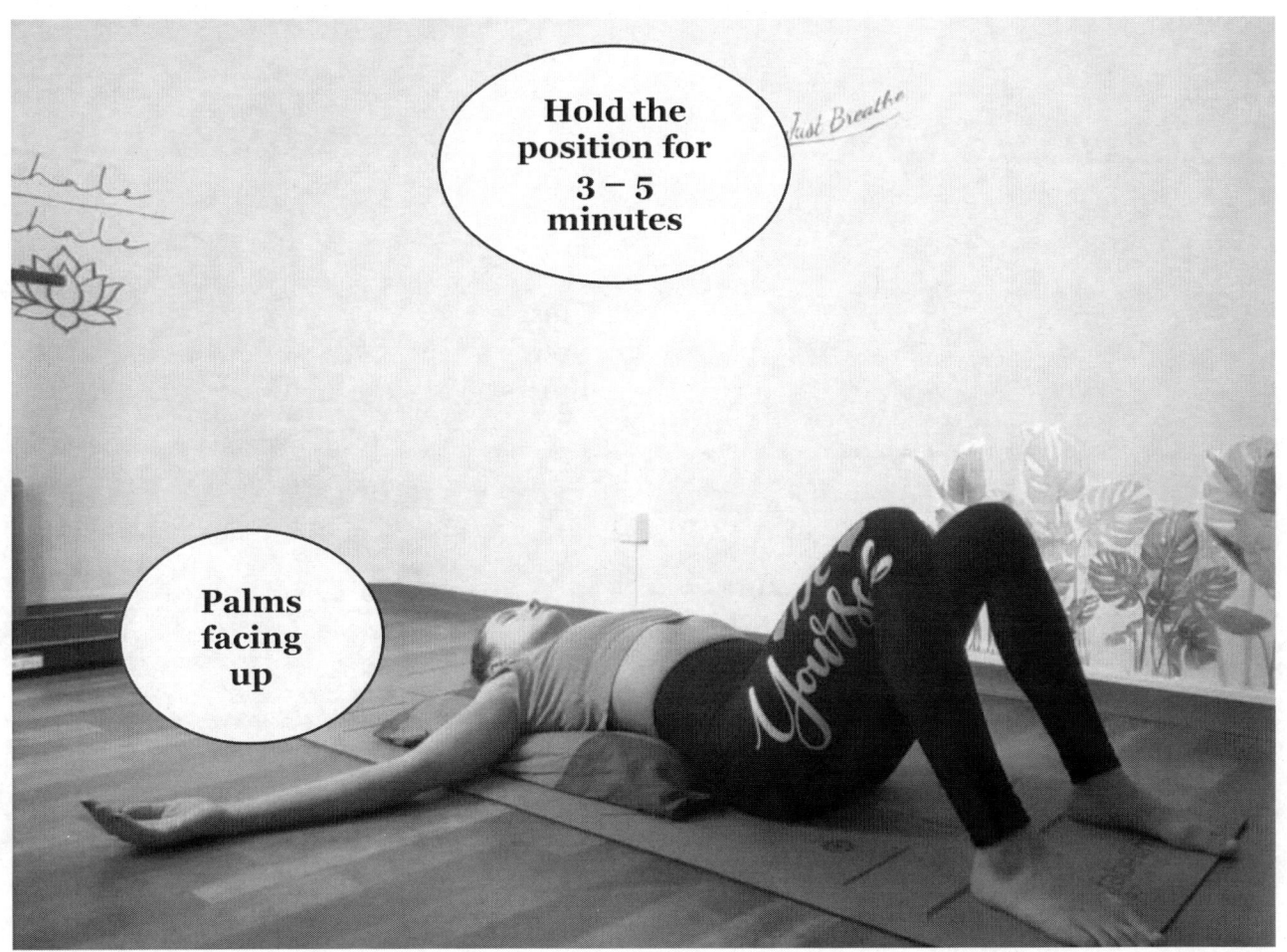

Hold the position for 3 – 5 minutes

Palms facing up

Manage Sorrow

Benefits

This somatic exercise helps to manage feelings of sorrow, providing a healthy outlet for emotional expression by working directly with the body.

Instructions

1. Stand straight with your back flat and feet hip width apart.

Breathing

Inhale and lengthen your spine with elbows wide.

Exhale and bring your chin to your chest, closing up your elbows.

Repetitions, Sets, and Rest

10 repetitions moving with your breath.

Suitable for

Manage feelings of sorrow.

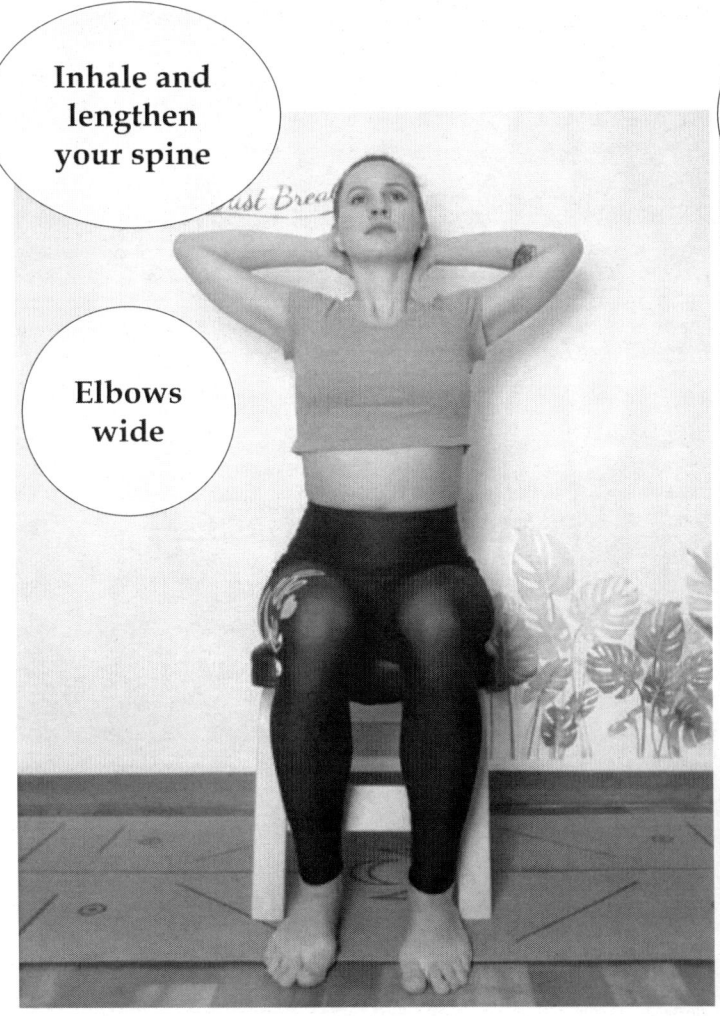

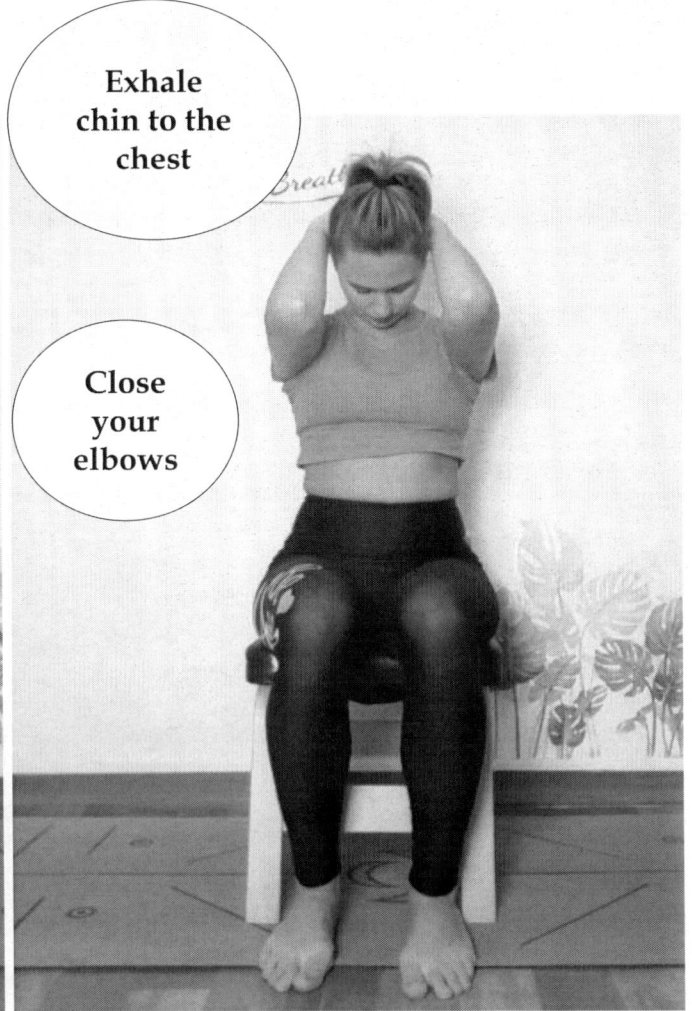

Manage Anxiety

Benefits

This exercise helps to activate the body's relaxation response, reducing the overall levels of stress and anxiety. This is achieved through a deep breathing, and gentle movements, which help calm the nervous system.

Instructions

1. Lie down on your belly. Preferably on your bed for more comfort. Legs extended and slightly apart from each other.

2. Rest your forehead on tops of your hands. Now rock your hips for 1 minute. Pause for 20 seconds.

Breathing

Breath normally during the exercise.

Repetitions, Sets, and Rest

Repeat the hips rock rocks 5 times.

Suitable for

Stress reduction.

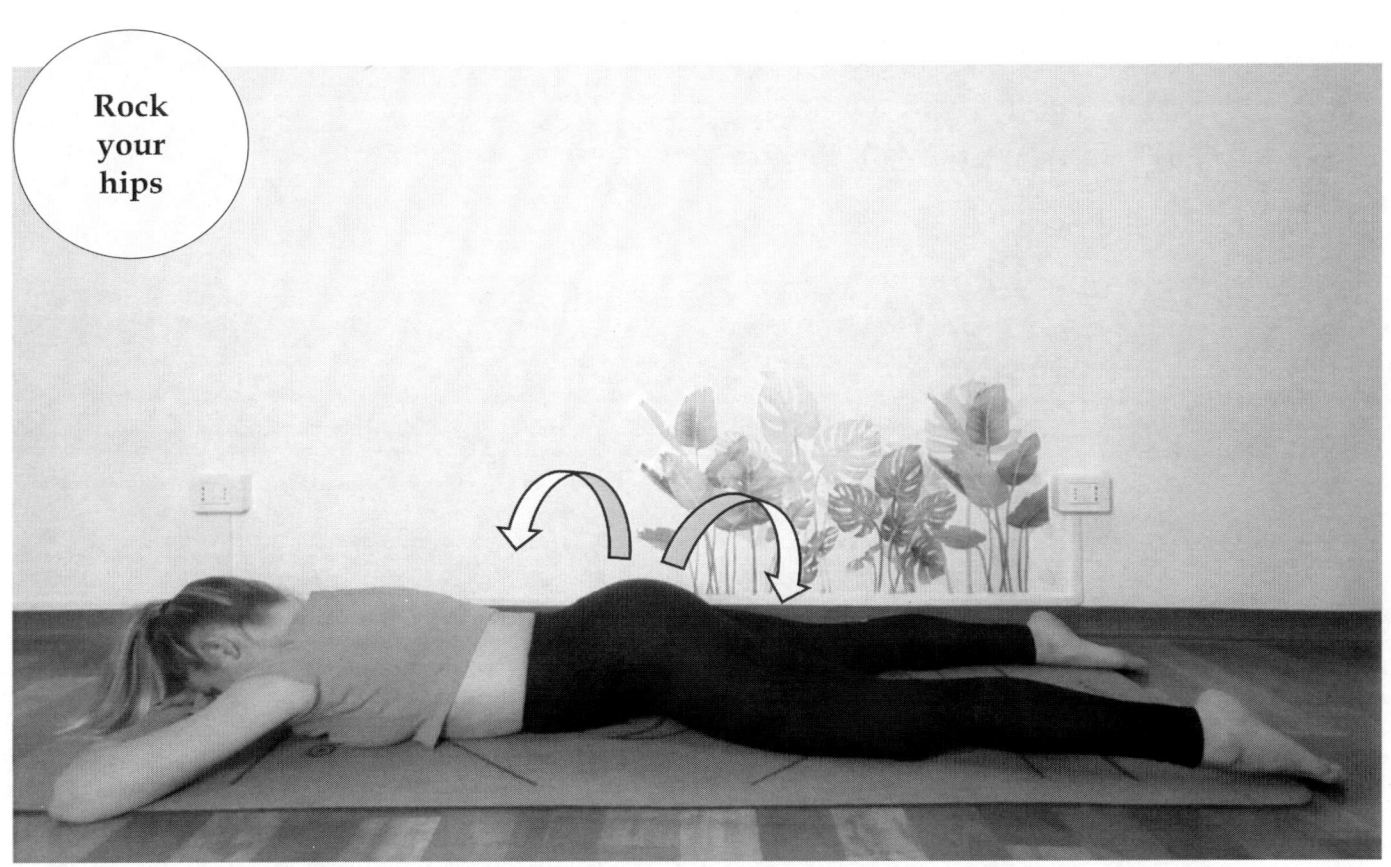

Rock your hips

Manage Fear

Benefits

Fear often manifests physically in the body through symptoms like increased heart rate, tension in the muscles, or shallow breathing. This exercise focuses on reduce these physical symptoms by promoting relaxation and releasing muscle tension.

Instructions

1. Lie on your left side, with a pillow under your head and your right arm extended on the floor. Knees slightly bend.

2. Rotate your head and left arm in parallel. Move your left arm forward 180 degrees at shoulder height, starting with your left hand touching your right hand and ending with it on the floor to your left.

3. Execute the exercise in the opposite side.

Breathing

Inhale to close your arms.

Exhale as you open up your arms.

Repetitions, Sets, and Rest

10 repetitions each side.

Suitable for

Reduce the stress and feelings of fear.

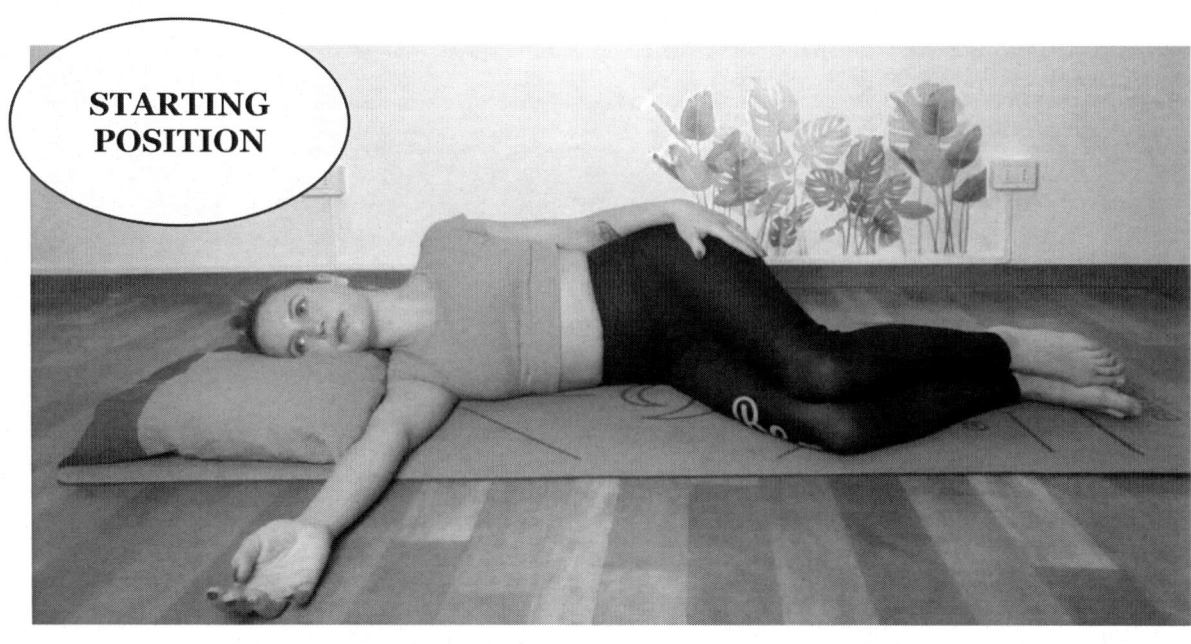

STARTING POSITION

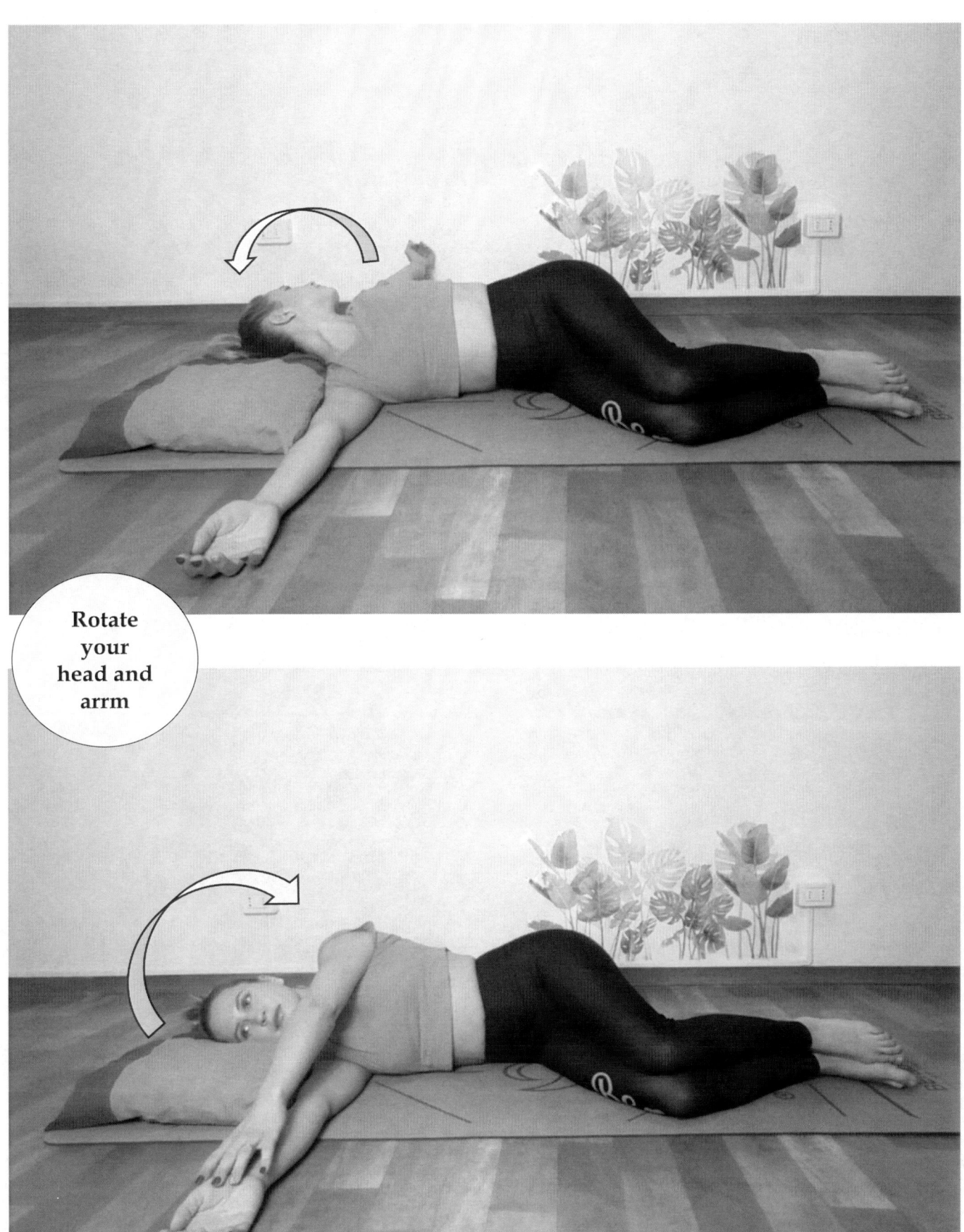

Rotate
your
head and
arrm

Manage Anger

Benefits

Anger often leads to physical tension in the body, particularly in areas like the jaw, neck, shoulders, and fists. Following exercise releases this tension, leading to a feeling of physical relaxation and emotional release.

Instructions

1. Stand tall with your legs a bit wider than your hips. Now bend from your hips into a forward fold. Place your hands flat on the floor.

2. Micro -bend one knee at a time. Repeat with the other leg.

Breathing

Normally breathe during the exercise.

Repetitions, Sets, and Rest

10 repetitions on each side for 1 to 2 sets, with 30 seconds rest between each set.

Suitable for

Reduce physical tension in the jaw, neck, shoulders and fists.

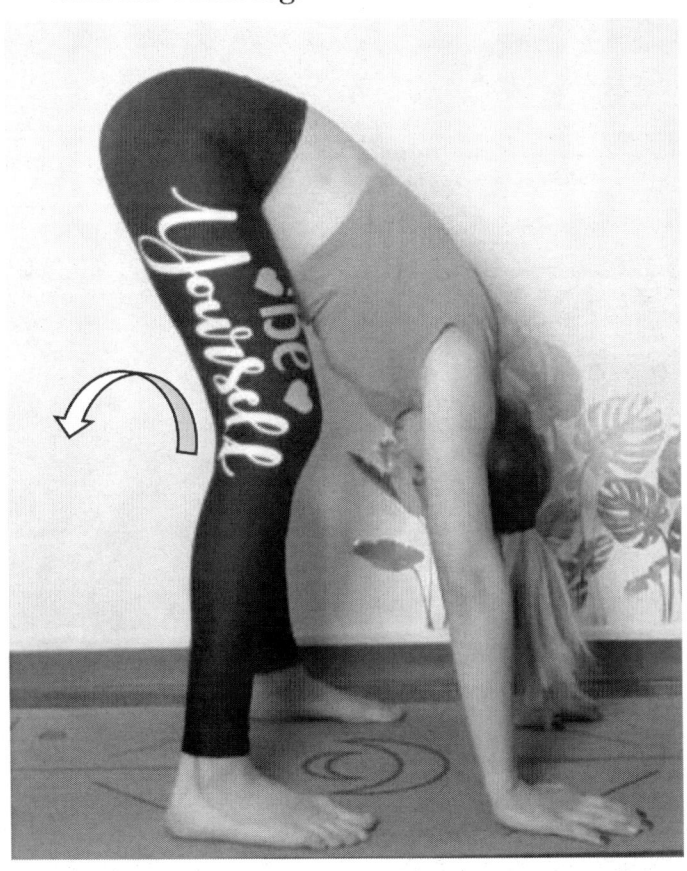
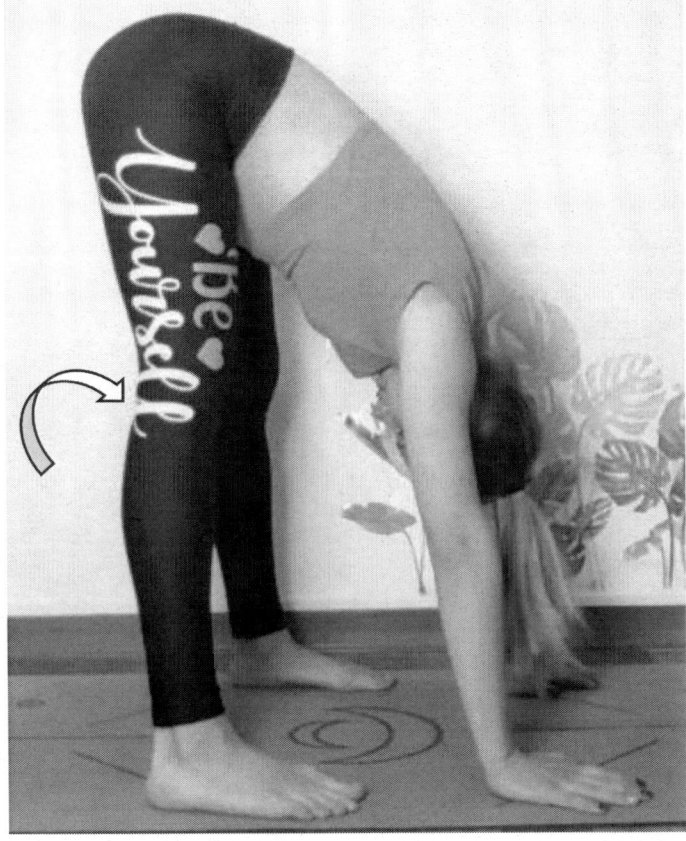

Manage Grief

Benefits

Grief can manifest physically in the body as tension or blocked energy. This exercise facilitates the release of these emotions, allowing for catharsis and a sense of relief from the intensity of grief.

Instructions

1. Lie on your back with your legs straight and slightly apart. Arms relaxed by your sides, but not too close to your body, palms facing down.

2. Gently rock your feet on the floor for 1 minute and pause for 20 seconds. Repeat the cycle 5 times.

Breathing

Inhale while stepping forward.

Exhale to lift up the knee.

Repetitions, Sets, and Rest

5 repetitions for 1 minute, resting for 20 seconds each cycle.

Suitable for

Release tension and blocked energy.

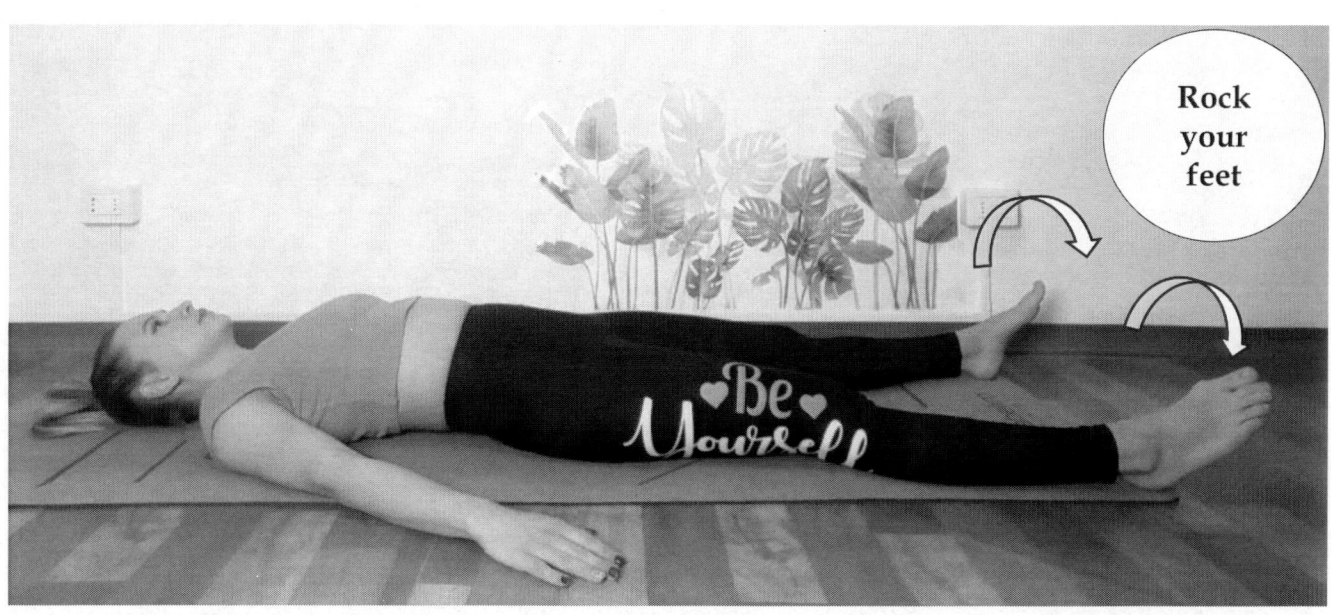

Rock your feet

Manage Panic and Panic attacks

Benefits

This exercise helps to develop a deeper understanding of your bodily sensations and how to regulate them to reduce panic symptoms.

Instructions

1. Sit onto your heels. Open up your knees and melt your chest down towards the floor. Extend your arms and cross your wrist on top of the other.

2. Rest your forehead on the mat. Hold for 5 breaths on both sides.

Breathing

Gently and deeply breath during the exercise.

Repetitions, Sets, and Rest

5 breaths each side.

Suitable for

Managing panic, increase body awareness, develop coping skills for emotional and physical regulation, and ultimately gain a greater sense of control over panic symptoms.

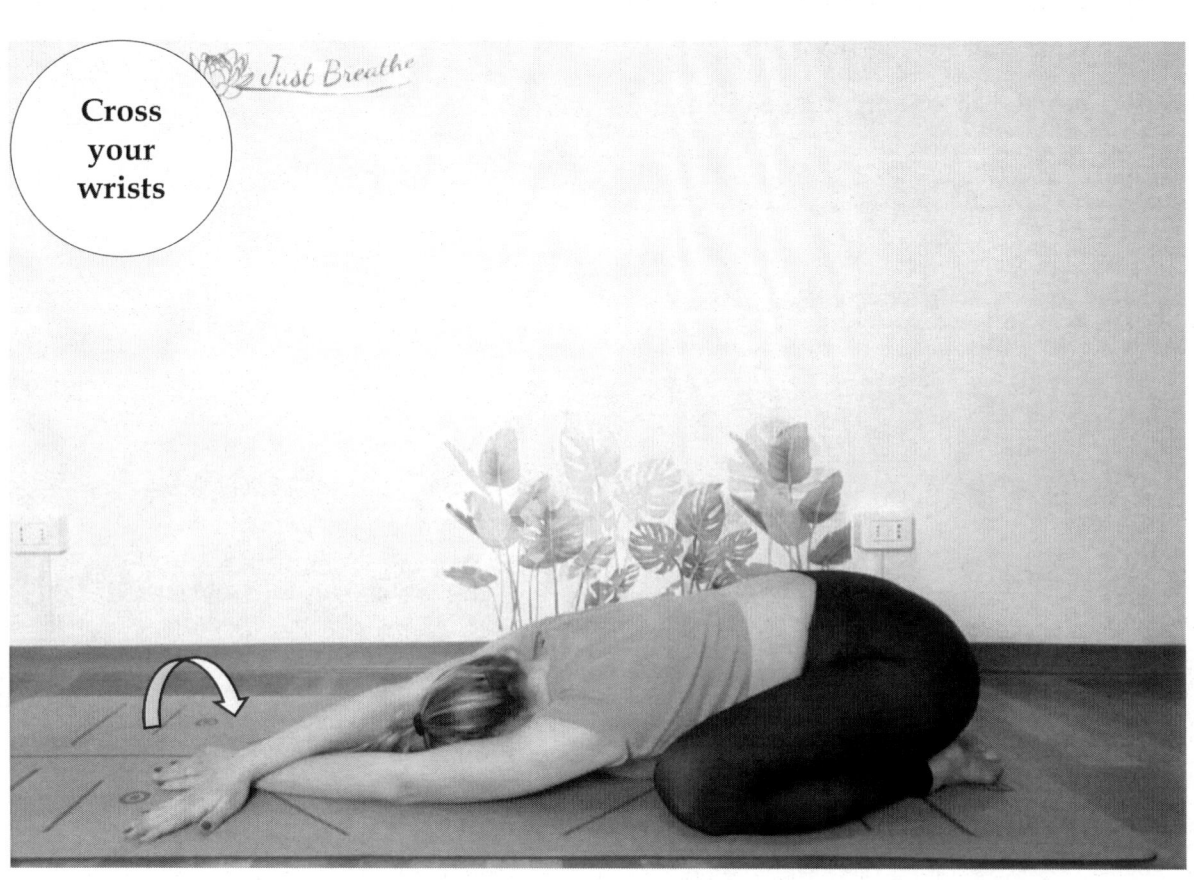

Manage the lack of Energy/ Overwhelmed

Benefits

This exercise helps to increase blood flow and oxygenation throughout the body, resulting in a boost in energy. In parallel it activated the body's relaxation response, reducing stress hormones such as cortisol. levels.

Instructions

1. Sit comfortably on your chair or on the floor. With your fingers, pull up your ears and nod your head gently up and down.

Breathing

Inhale as you nod your head up.

Exhale as you nod your head down.

Repetitions, Sets, and Rest

8 repetitions.

Suitable for

Boost energy and activate the body's relaxation response.

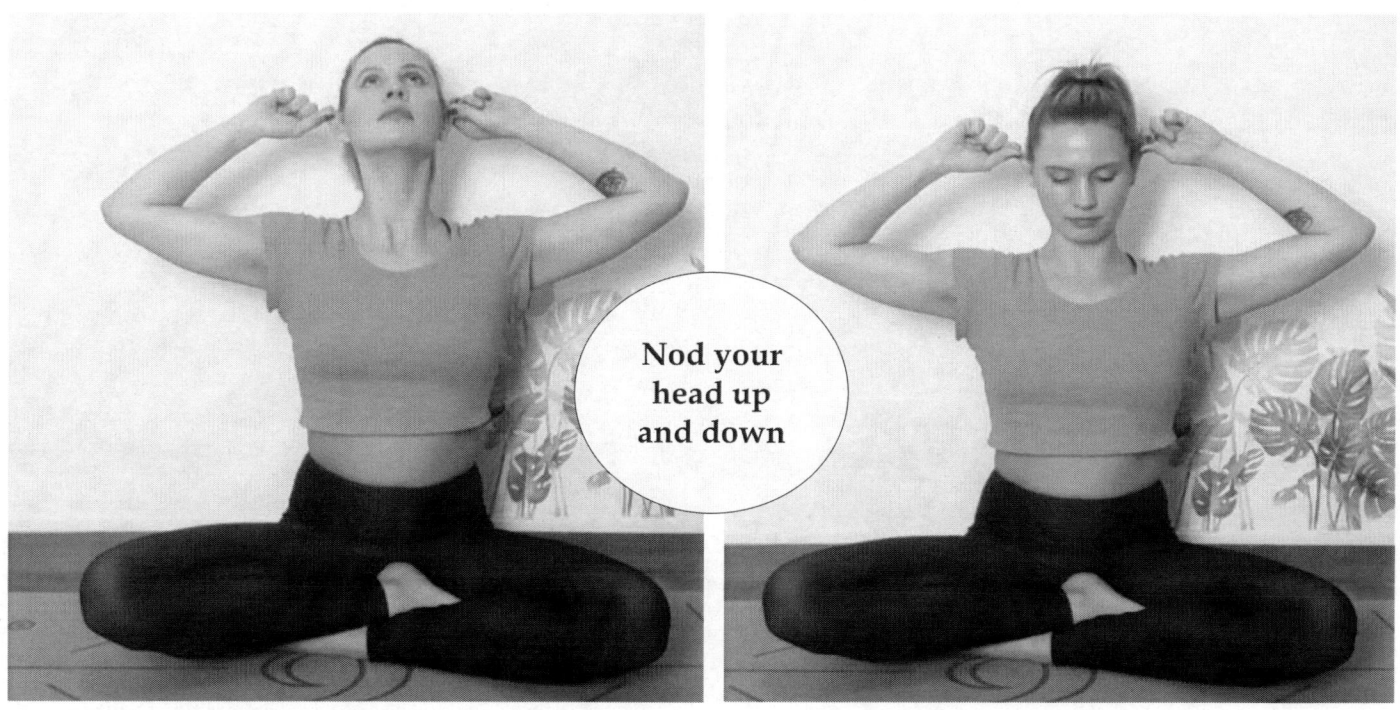

Nod your head up and down

Wipe Away difficult emotions

Benefits

This exercise is highly recommended for driving away difficult emotions and clearing the mind of negative thoughts.

Instructions

1. Stand tall with your feet slightly wider than your hips.

2. Bend over to a position that feels good for your body.

3. Sweep your arms from side to side and wipe away whatever frustrations you have.

Breathing

Normally breath during the exercise.

Repetitions, Sets, and Rest

Sweep your arms for 30 – 60 seconds.

Suitable for

Wipe away all your frustrations.

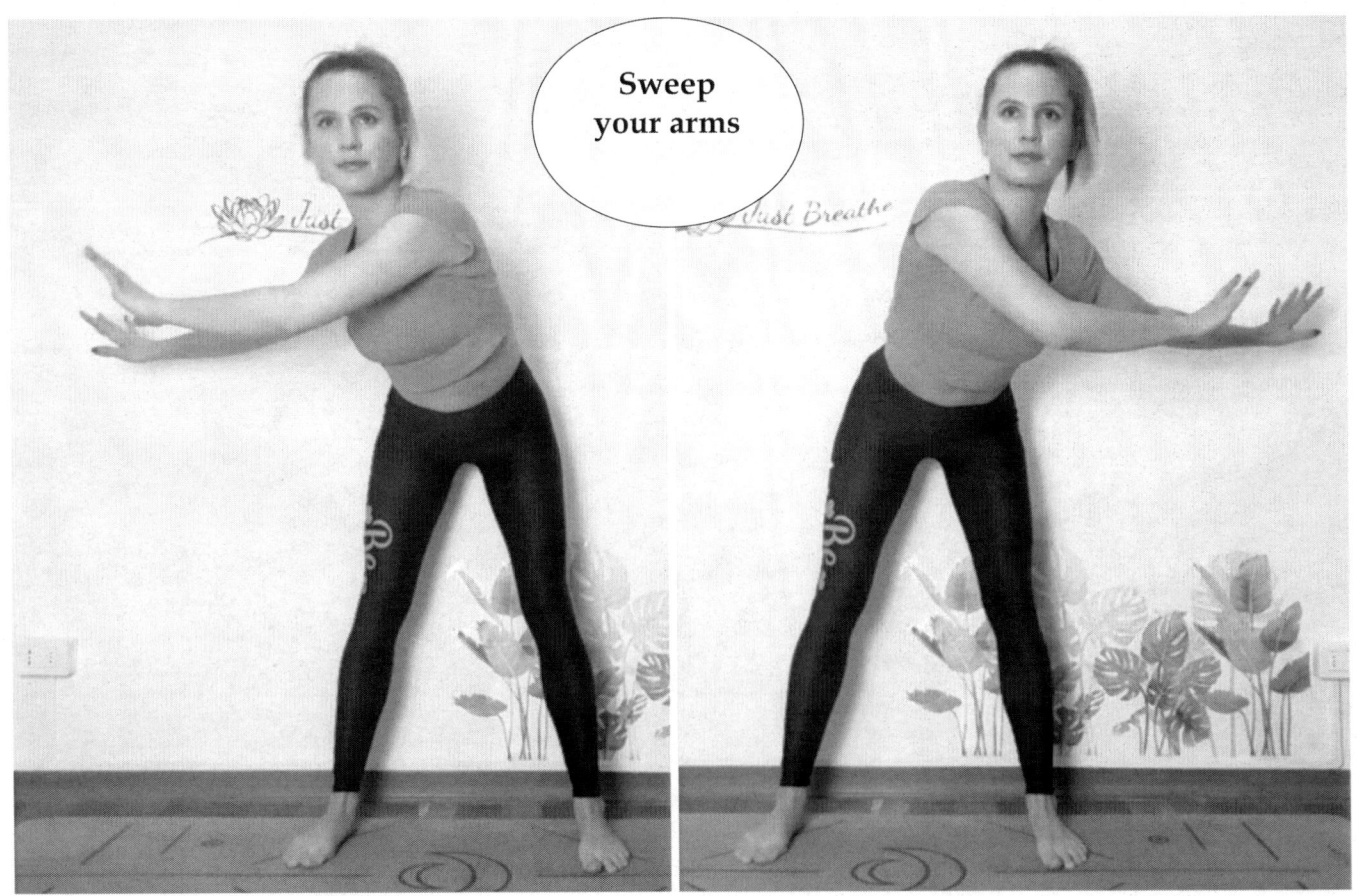

Sweep your arms

Release positive emotions: Butterfly Hug

Benefits

This exercise evokes positive emotions, such as joy, gratitude, or love, leading to an immediate improvement in mood.

Instructions

1. Stand or sit in a comfortable position. Interlace your thumbs fingers wide and bring your hands across your chest.

2. Let your fingers reach towards your shoulders. Allow yourself to settle in, feeling the comfort and that soothing sensation of your arms.

3. When you feel ready, gently alternate your fingers, by tapping them onto your shoulders, whatever feels good for you.

Breathing

Deeply breath during the exercise.

Repetitions, Sets, and Rest

Practice this exercise as log as you need.

Suitable for

Mood enhancement

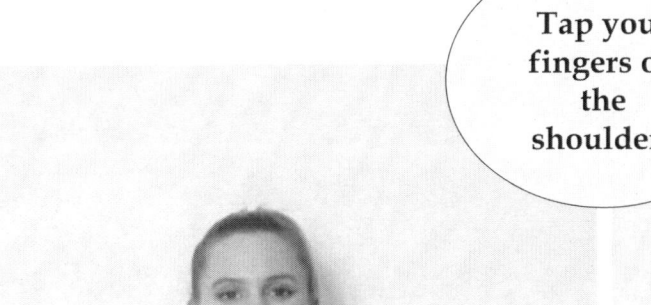

Tap your fingers on the shoulders

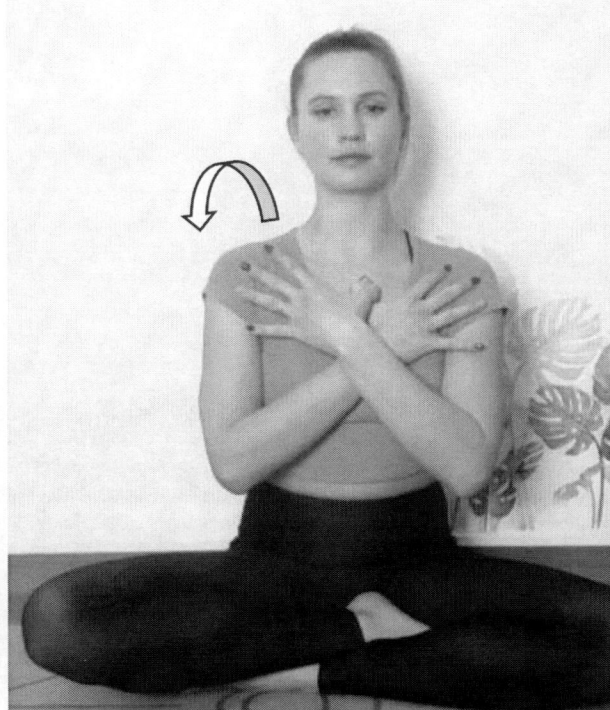

Release positive emotions: Goddess

Benefits

This exercise helps you experience feelings of happiness and contentment.

Instructions

1. Stand tall, feet apart and your toes turned out. Bring your palms in prayer position in front of your chest.

2. Squat down, then go up and reach your arms towards the ceiling.

TIPS

Do the exercise at a pace that feels good for you.

Breathing

Inhale to squat down.

Exhale to go up.

Repetitions, Sets, and Rest

10 repetitions for 1 -2 sets, resting 30 seconds each set.

Suitable for

Experience feelings of happiness and contentment.

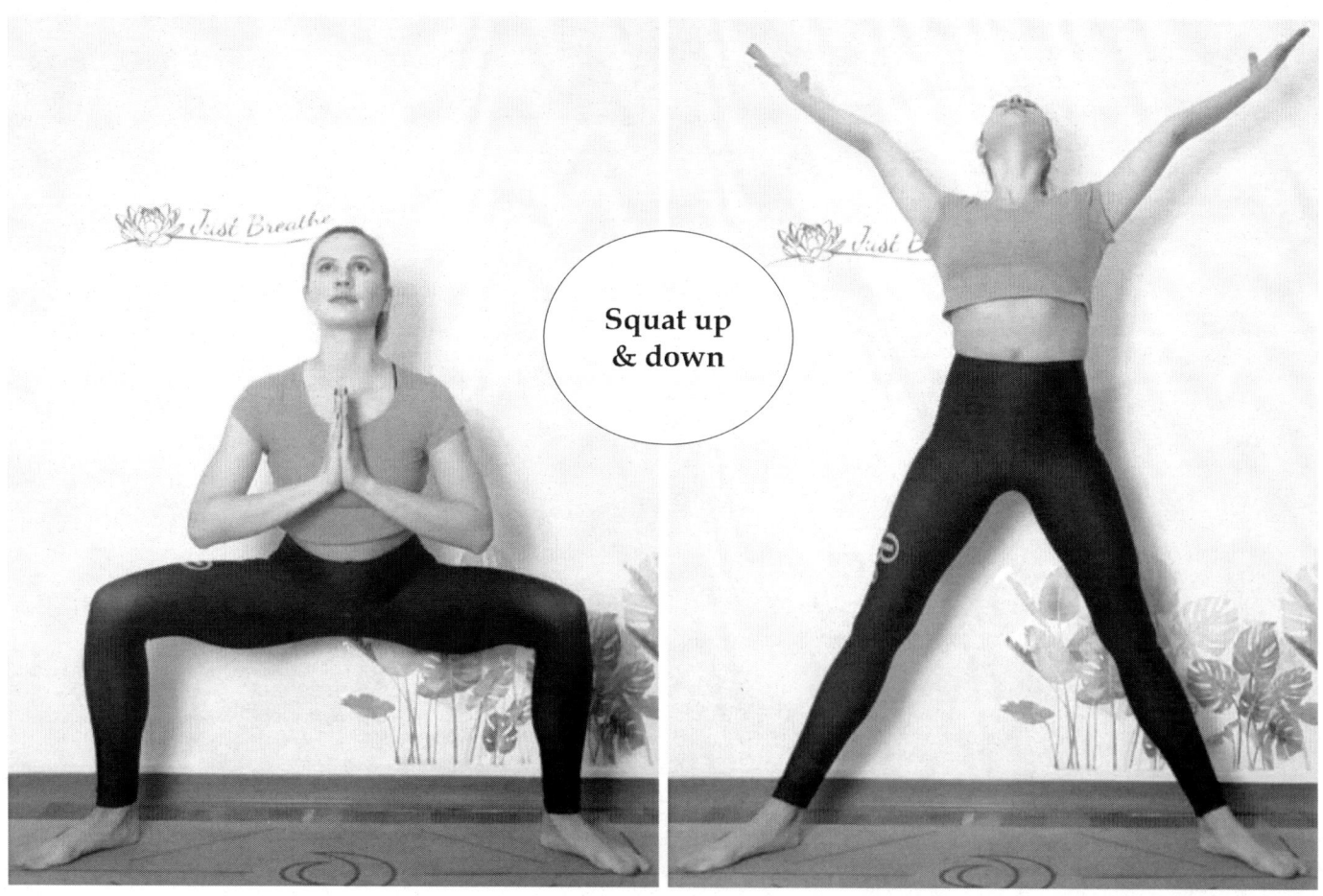

Squat up & down

Chapter 7: Somatic Exercises for Mindfulness

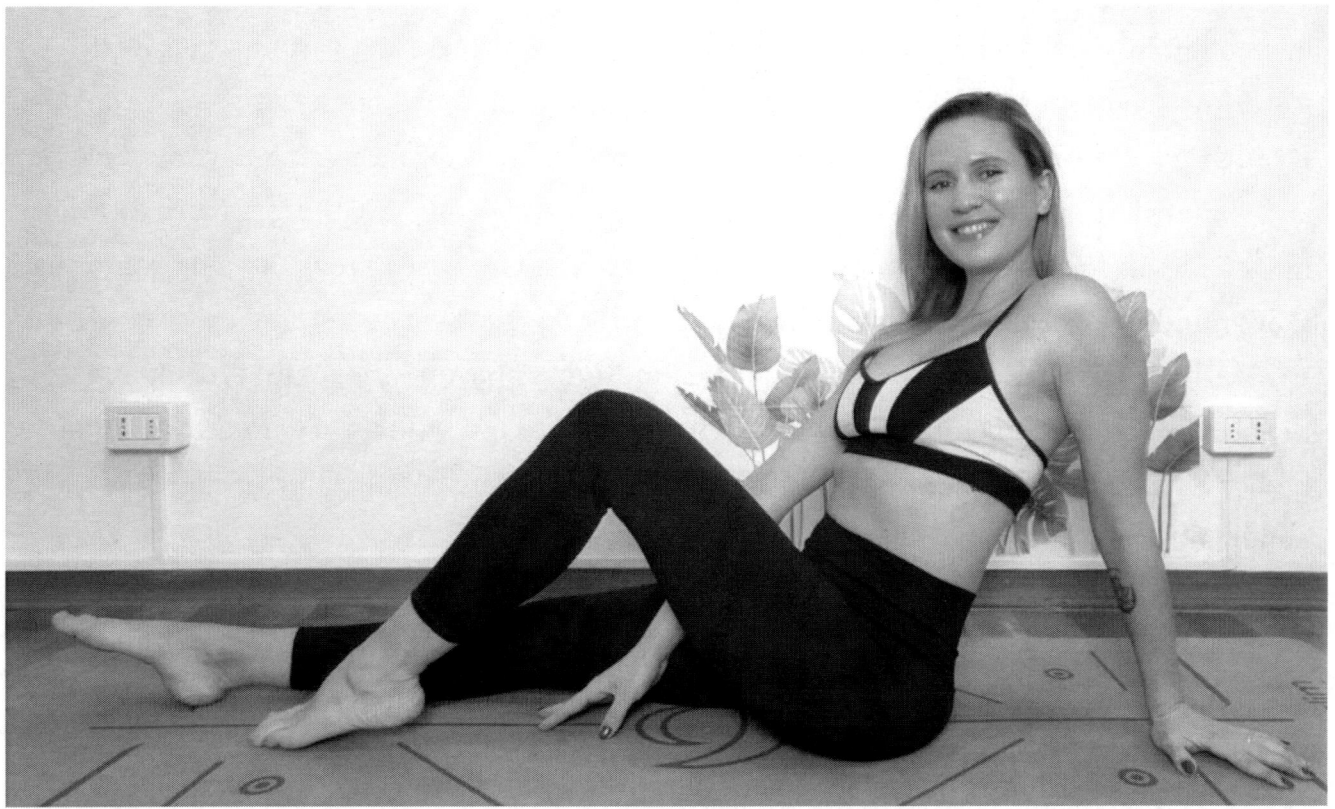

The Mind-Body Link in Somatic and Mindfulness

The *Mindfulness* word has recently been included in Western psychology and medicine but is a very old technique that dates back more than 2,500 years and forms the core of Buddhist teachings. The connection between mindfulness and somatics is deep-rooted, as both practices share a fundamental focus on cultivating awareness, presence, and an intimate understanding of the mind-body connection. Here are several key aspects that highlight the connection between mindfulness and somatics:

1. **Present-Moment Awareness:** Mindfulness involves being fully present in the current moment, and somatics similarly encourages present-moment awareness. In somatic practices, individuals are guided to direct their attention inward, fostering a heightened awareness of bodily sensations, movement patterns, and emotional states.

2. **Body Sensation Awareness:** Both mindfulness and somatics place a strong emphasis on paying attention to bodily sensations. In somatic exercises, individuals are encouraged to explore and observe the subtle sensations, tensions, or releases within the body. This heightened awareness facilitates a deeper understanding of one's physical state.

3. **Mindful Movement:** Mindful movement is a common thread between mindfulness and somatics. In both practices, movements are intentional, slow, and purposeful. Mindful movement in somatics involves exploring how the body feels during various exercises, fostering a conscious and deliberate engagement with each movement.

4. **Breath Awareness:** Mindfulness often incorporates breath awareness as a central element, and somatics similarly emphasizes the importance of conscious breathing. Breath awareness in somatics serves as a tool for relaxation, facilitating the release of tension and promoting a more mindful engagement with the body.

5. **Embodied Mindfulness:** Somatics takes mindfulness beyond the mental realm and into the body, making it an embodied practice. It encourages individuals to connect with their bodies on a deep level, exploring how thoughts and emotions manifest physically. This embodied mindfulness is a distinctive feature of somatics.

6. **Release of Tension and Stress:** Both mindfulness and somatics aim to reduce tension and stress in the body. Mindfulness practices, including meditation and mindful breathing, contribute to stress reduction, and somatics achieves a similar outcome by promoting awareness and release of habitual muscular tension.

7. **Mind-Body Integration:** Mindfulness and Somatic promote the integration of the mind and body. In somatics, the term "somatic" refers to the unity of the mind and body as a holistic entity. The practices encourage individuals to recognize and address the interconnectedness of mental and physical well-being.

8. **Non-Judgmental Observation:** Mindfulness emphasizes non-judgmental observation of thoughts and feelings, and somatics extends this approach to the body. Individuals practicing somatics are encouraged to observe bodily sensations without judgment, fostering self-compassion and acceptance.

9. **Enhanced Body Awareness:** Both mindfulness and somatics contribute to enhanced body awareness. Through somatic practices, individuals develop a deep understanding of their bodies' patterns, movements, and responses, leading to increased self-awareness.

The connection between mindfulness and somatic is evident in their shared philosophy of embracing the present moment, cultivating awareness, and recognizing the intricate relationship between the mind and body. As individuals engage in somatic practices with a mindful approach, they can experience profound benefits for both physical and mental well-being.

Mindfulness-based movement practices, such as Tai Chi and Qigong, focus on cultivating awareness of the body in motion.

Exercise 1: Somatic Meditation

Benefits

This exercise heightens awareness of your body, fosters mindfulness by grounding you in the present moment, and cultivates a deeper connection with bodily experiences.

Instructions

1. Sit comfortably and start by asking yourself, "What has your attention right now?" Focus on sensory awareness rather than your thoughts. Tune into your senses, noticing what you see, hear, feel, and any sensations in your body.

2. Observe your surroundings, allowing your gaze to land on objects that draw your attention. Maintain connection with your external environment while focusing on internal sensations. You can close your eyes or keep them open with a soft gaze lowered a few feet in front.

3. Rest your hands on your knees with palms facing down for grounding, up for receiving. Bring attention to the physical sensations inside your body. Start by feeling into your hands, fingers, and palms. There are no right sensations; just explore the effects of conscious contact.

4. Slowly shift your attention to different regions of your body.

Breathing

Gently breath during the meditation.

Repetitions, Sets, and Rest

Whenever you want throughout the day.

Suitable for

Boost the awareness of your body.

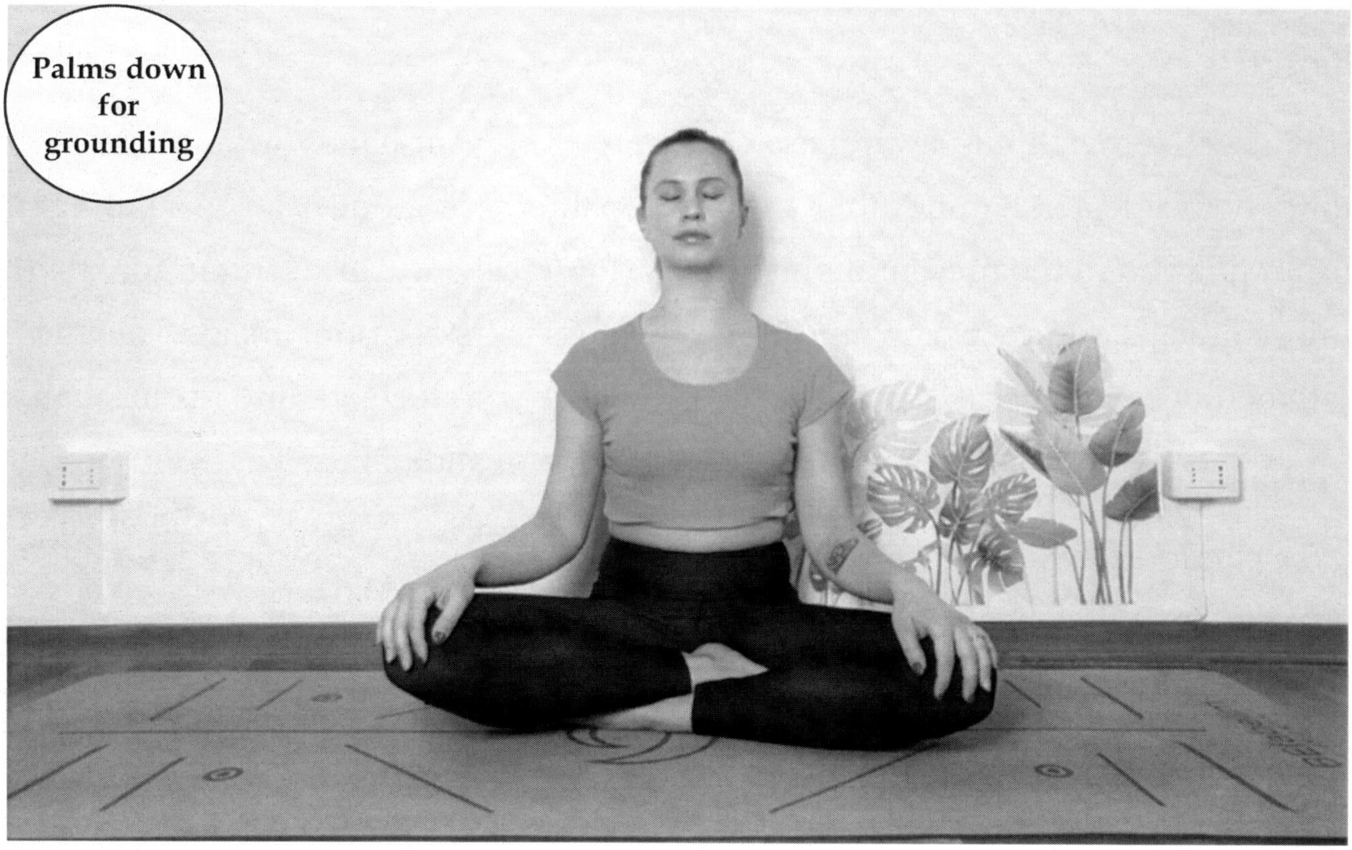

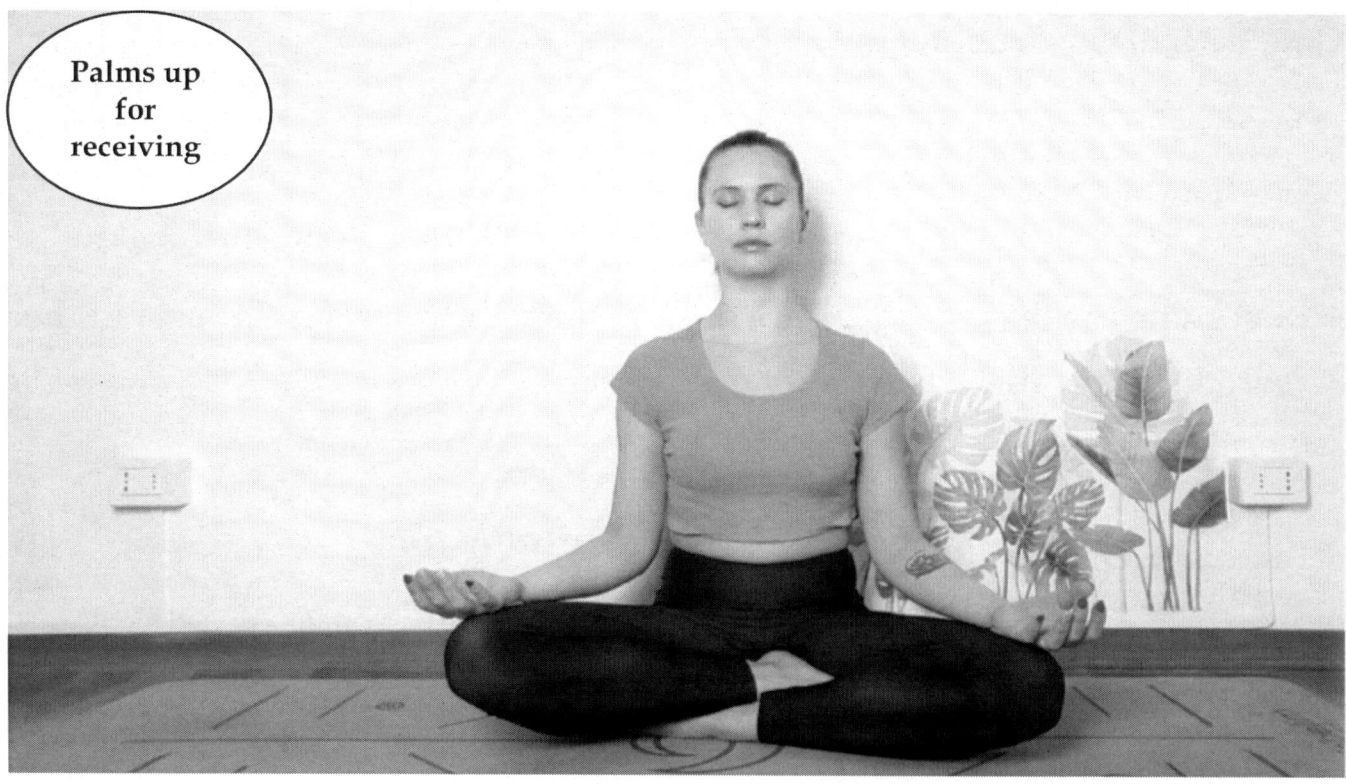

Palms down for grounding

Palms up for receiving

Exercise 2: Find your Feet

Benefits

This exercise heightens sensory awareness in your feet. This increased sensitivity allows you to notice subtle sensations, textures, and movements, promoting a deeper connection with your body and recharge your energy after a tough day of work... maybe spent on heels.

Instructions

1. Sit on a chair or stand on the ground. You can do this exercise with your socks or barefoot. Close your eyes, breathe, and relax.

2. Start with one foot and wiggle your toes. Roll your toes from big toe to your pinky. Notice what they feel like: are they cold, hot, tight or loose?

3. Press your heel firmly into the ground for a moment and then release.

4. Switch your attention to your other foot, roll and wiggle your toes. Notice the same thing as the other foot: are they sore or relaxed? light or heavy?

5. Press your heel into the ground and lift your foot up. Feel the nice stretch. Now bring attention to both of your feet. How do they feel? There is no right or wrong.

Breathing

Gently breath during the meditation.

Repetitions, Sets, and Rest

Whenever you want throughout the day.

Suitable for

Sensory awareness and energy recharging for your feet.

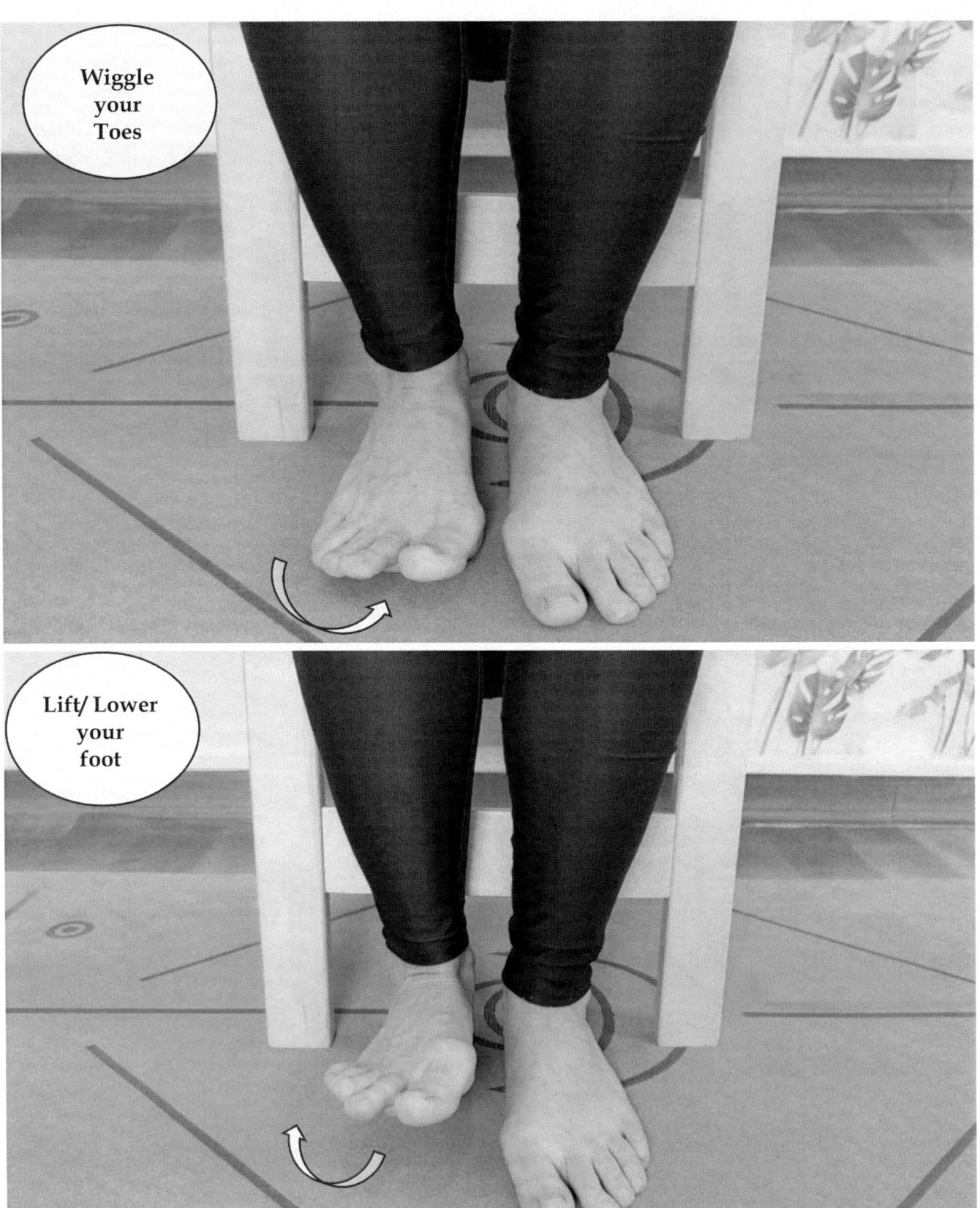

BONUS CHAPTER: Somatic Exercise to lose belly

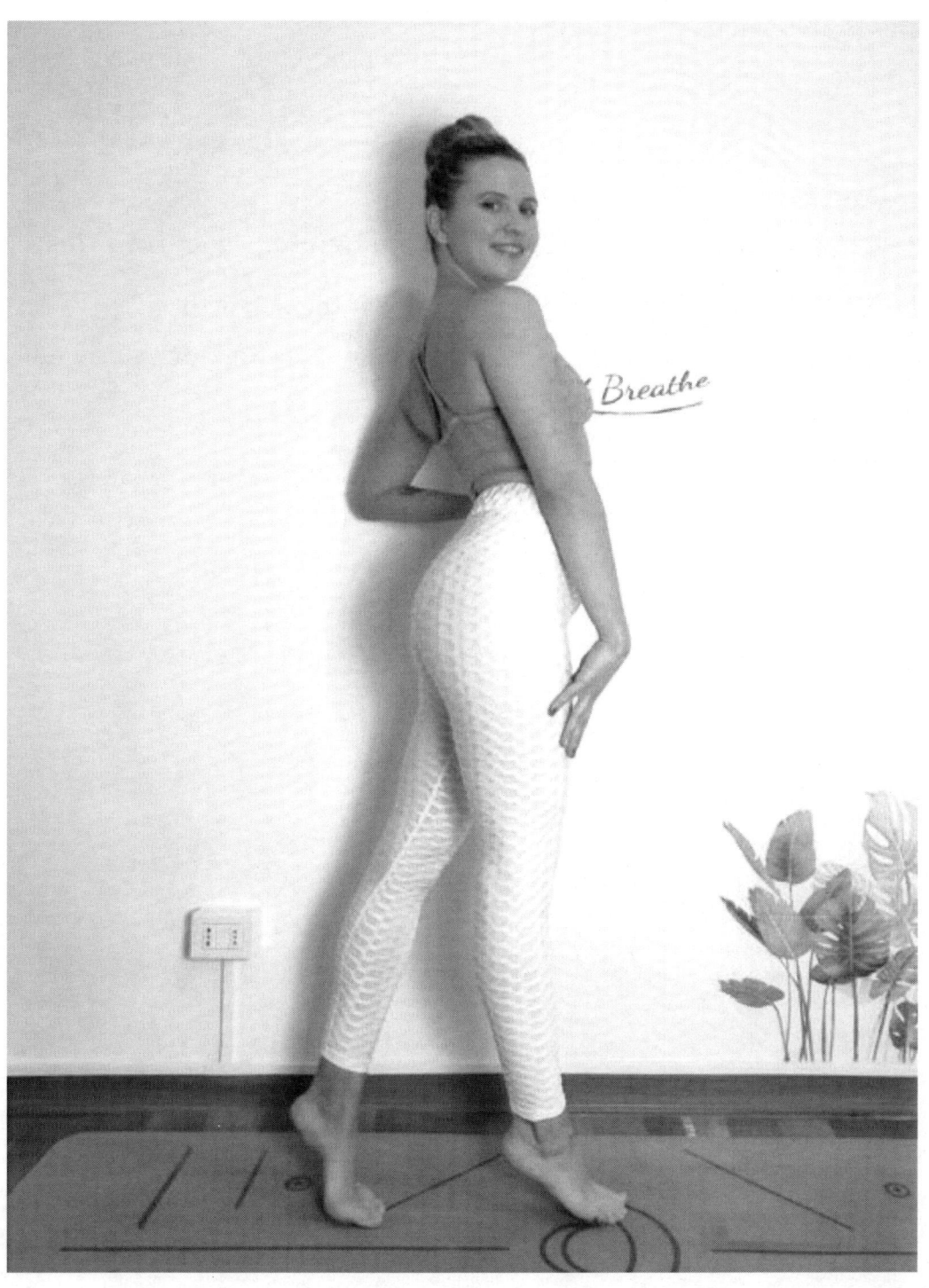

Benefits

To lose weight in your belly, you need stop high intensity workouts for 1 Month and release the stress & trauma out of your body first. Practice this exercise in parallel with the Somatic Exercises for Release Trauma

Instructions

1. Lie on your back, knees bent and feet hip distance apart, arms by your sides not too close to your body and palms facing down.

2. tilt your pelvis up and down, engaging your core muscles. Flatten your back against the floor by tightening your abdominal muscles and bending your pelvis up slightly.

3. curve your back slightly and tilt your pelvis down towards the ground.

Breathing

Deeply Inhale and Exhale 2-3 times before starting the exercise.

Inhale as you tilt your pelvis up

Exhale as you tilt your pelvis down.

Repetitions, Sets, and Rest

Repeat the pelvis tilt for 30 – 60 seconds for 5 sets, resting for 20 seconds between each set.

Suitable for

Lose belly fat.

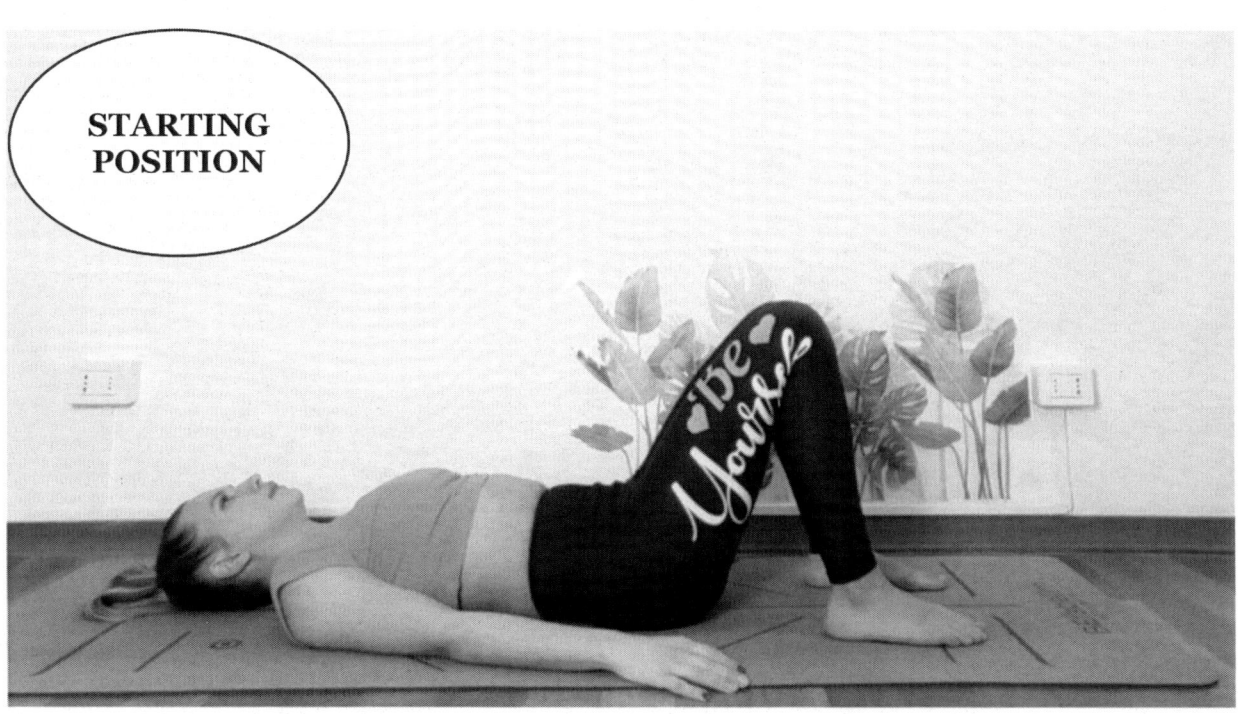

STARTING POSITION

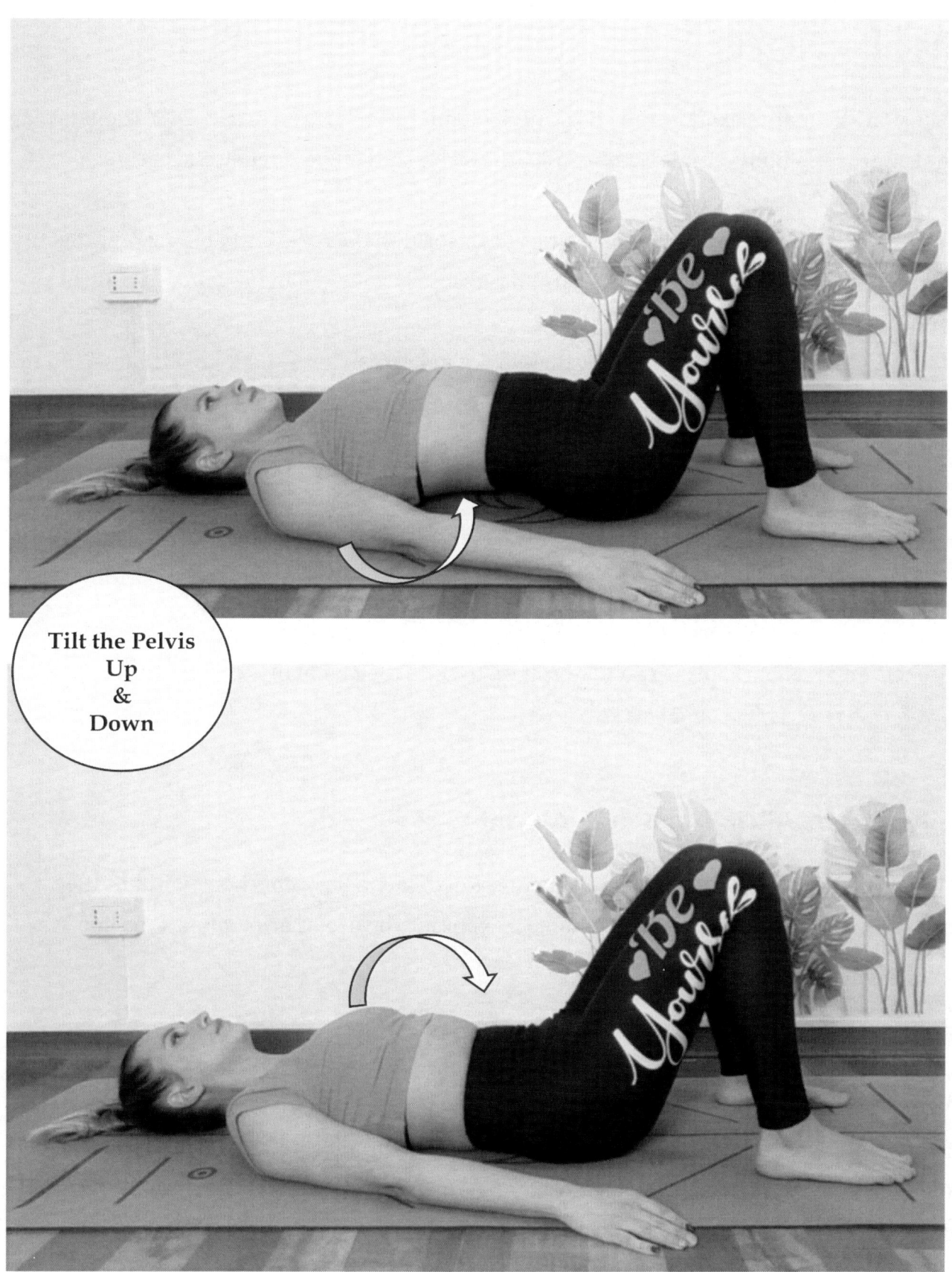

Tilt the Pelvis
Up
&
Down

Conclusion

In conclusion, "Somatics exercises for Beginners" is not just a book; it's a 28-DAY transformative journey towards the Body-Mind reconnection, the stress and anxiety relief, the chronic pain reduction, and weight loss.

The Benefits of Somatics are truly remarkable. In a world that rushes and no longer grants time for oneself, in just a few minutes a day, you can rediscover yourself and regain full control of your mind and body.

If you've found this book enjoyable and valuable, I'd like to ask for a small favor that would make a huge impact. **An honest and opened review on Amazon** would be truly invaluable. Reader opinions like yours not only help me grow as an author but also assist other readers in their choice. Below, based on your country, you can find the link to leave the review:

US: https://www.amazon.com/review/create-review/?asin=B0CWBJDQ5B

UK: https://www.amazon.co.uk/review/create-review/?asin= B0CWBJDQ5B

CA: https://www.amazon.ca/review/create-review/?asin= B0CWBJDQ5B

For contacts and feedback, please do not hesitate to send me an email at:

aliciadiamond.fitness@gmail.com

Alicia

Disclaimer:

The information and exercises provided in this book are for educational purposes only and should not be considered a substitute for professional medical advice. This book does not constitute professional medical guidance, diagnosis, or treatment. It is strongly recommended to consult a doctor or qualified healthcare provider before starting any new fitness program or making changes to an existing one, included the fitness program reported in present book.

The author and publisher are not liable for any injuries, health issues, or adverse effects resulting from the application of the methods described in this book. The reader bears full responsibility for their health and safety.

Manufactured by Amazon.ca
Acheson, AB

13695864R00063